SUPERSTITION
IN MEDICINE

WWW.THEOPHANIA.CA

© 2014, Theophania Publishing.

SUPERSTITION
IN MEDICINE

BY

PROF. DR. HUGO MAGNUS

AUTHORIZED TRANSLATION FROM
THE GERMAN, EDITED BY

Dr. JULIUS L. SALINGER

*Late Assistant Professor of Clinical Medicine, Jefferson Medical
College; Physician to the Philadelphia General Hospital, etc.*

PREFACE

The history of medicine is closely interlinked with the development of theology. The errors of one are for the most part reflected in the mistakes of the other. No matter how obscure and dark the origin of either, whether derived from ignorance and superstition or not, the ultimate achievement alone must be taken into consideration. We do not reject chemistry because it originated in alchemy, we do not disregard astronomy because its roots are entwined with the teachings of astrology, and so in theology and medicine we look to the final issue. The statements set forth in this book should not be construed as reflecting the development of theology or medicine at the time, but as the belief of the people existing in these periods. Philosophy may have been pure, but if the mind of man was faulty the responsibility must not be laid at the door of science. It is the function of the historian truthfully to depict the thought and spirit of the time of which he writes. This has been attempted in the present work. It is not a criticism of a system, but a criticism of man. There can be no doubt that absurd superstitions are still existent for which the twentieth century will be severely criticized in time to come. Thus the words of our martyred President may well be used as a motto for this book: "With malice towards none, with charity for all."

The last chapter of this book has been added by the translator, as it seemed necessary for the full discussion of the subject.

JULIUS L. SALINGER.

PHILADELPHIA, Pa.

I

WHAT IS MEDICAL SUPERSTITION?

FAITH and superstition are twin brothers. Altho the former leads humanity to its sublimest ideals and the latter only presents us with a caricature of human knowledge, both are children of the same family. Both originate in a sense of the inadequacy of human science in regard to natural phenomena. The fact that the most important processes of organic life can not be traced to their ultimate origin, but that their investigation will soon lead to a point of irresistible opposition to further analysis, has always called forth a feeling of impotency and dependence in the human mind. This consciousness of being dependent upon factors which are entirely beyond human understanding has thus given rise to the metaphysical need of reflecting upon these mysterious factors, and bringing them within reach of human comprehension. Humanity, in attempting to satisfy such a metaphysical requirement from an ethical standpoint, created faith, which subsequently found expression in the various forms of religion. It is not within the scope of this essay to consider how far Divine revelations have been vouchsafed on this subject. Superstition undoubtedly entered the scene when, simultaneously with these, endeavors were made to consider and to explain physical processes from the standpoint of such metaphysical requirements. It is true that this did not, at first, lead to a marked contrast between faith and superstition; for a period existed in which faith and superstition—i.e., the metaphysical consideration of ethical values and the metaphysical consideration of the entire phenomena of life—were not only equivalent, but even merged into one conception. This occurred in an age in which mankind considered all terrestrial processes, whether they were of a psychical or of a material nature, as immediately caused by the steady interference of supernatural powers—a period during which the deity was held responsible for all terrestrial phenomena. During this period faith became superstition, and superstition, faith. A separation did not take place until some especially enlightened minds began to evolve the idea that it would be more reasonable to explain natural phenomena—temporal becoming, being, and passing away—by natural rather than by supernatural causes. The reaction against this better interpretation, the tenacious adherence to the original association of terrestrial manifestations with metaphysical factors, created the superstition of the natural sciences. The birth of superstition in the Greek world must be placed about the seventh century, B.C., the period during which Thales of Miletus came forward with his endeavor to explain natural processes in a natural manner. This attempt of the Milesian is the initiation of a rational scientific conception of natural manifestations, and the ancient theistic consideration of nature became superstition only in opposition to such a view. It follows, then, that what holds good with regard to the interpretation of natural manifestations in general holds good in medicine especially. Here, also, superstition came into question only when, besides the original theistic conception of the functions of the body and besides the metaphysical treatment of the sick, a valuation of the normal as well as of the morbid phenomena of the human organism came into vogue which took into account terrestrial causes. Not until this stage was reached did theism and theurgy lose their title and become superstition; until then they could claim fullest acceptance in medicine as thoroughly logical consequences of the prevailing theory of life. This took place, so far as Greek medicine was concerned, at about the end of the sixth century, B.C. The Corpus Hippocraticum already shows us Greek medicine as being purified from all theistic sophistications and only reckoning with natural causes. When this separation must have taken place for pre-Greek, Indian, Assyrian, and Egyptian culture can not be at present determined with certainty. For the Egyptian and Babylonico-Assyrian manuscripts, so far known, show an intimate admixture of true observation of nature with theistic speculations—i.e., a treatment of medicine which, altho it took account of physico-natural manifestations, was still deeply tinctured with superstition.

According to what we have stated, medical superstition might be defined as follows: "Belief that the normal as well as the pathological manifestations of organic life may be explained and eventually treated, without consideration of their physical nature, by means of supernatural agencies."

Medical superstition varies according to the kind and the origin of these supernatural causes, and therefore appears in the greatest variety of forms. If these causes were looked for in celestial regions, medical superstition became vested with the religious garb, and its source was in the religious cult; but if the belief prevailed that God shared the domination of the world with other mysterious elements, such as were embodied in different forms in accordance with the various philosophical systems, medical superstition bore a philosophical and mystical stamp whose origin is revealed in the history of philosophy. But if certain mysterious powers hidden in the womb of nature or active above the earth were considered to influence human life, medical superstition assumed a physical character. However, it frequently followed that the above three factors acted simultaneously or in varying combinations, or certain other elements which were inherent in human nature cooperated. For this reason it is sometimes not quite easy to decide as to the source from which this or that form of medical superstition principally derived its persistent currency. But, nevertheless, it is our intention to divide our subject in accordance with the sources from which the several forms of medical superstition spring, as it is absolutely impossible to obtain a satisfactory view of the extensive material without first attempting a systematic arrangement of the data at hand.

But before attempting to inquire why the purest and most valuable fountains of all human knowledge—religion, philosophy, and natural science—have at the same time become sources of medical superstition, it will be advisable to explain the character which medical science had assumed under the exclusive domination of theism, and how conditions shaped themselves when physico-mechanical philosophy appeared and began to do battle with the theistic conception of life. These conditions played such a special part in the development of medico-physical superstition that it becomes necessary first to examine their power and tendency before attempting to contemplate medical superstition proper.

II

THEISM IN ITS RELATION TO MEDICINE AND IN ITS STRUGGLE WITH THE PHYSICO-MECHANICAL THEORY OF LIFE

AS WE explained in Chapter I., the development of all peoples has passed through a period during which medico-physical knowledge found expression exclusively in the teachings of religion. By theism we mean the system which endeavors to explain natural phenomena by supernatural causes. However, this view of nature, with its tinge of religion, did not as yet show any trace of superstition. It was rather the only justifiable conception of nature and thoroughly in keeping with the power of comprehension of man, until it began to dawn upon the mind that natural phenomena might be due to natural causes. This was the period of which we stated, in the beginning of this investigation, that faith became superstition and superstition became faith. It was during this time that the powers above were held accountable for all bodily ailments of mankind. It was their task most carefully to observe the functional processes of the human body in all its phases, and to protect their undisturbed continuance. But as the inhabitants of heaven, like the inhabitants of the earth, were subject to whims, it happened very often, unfortunately, that they attended to their task of protecting the undisturbed development of the vegetative as well as the animal functions of the body in a very unsatisfactory manner, sometimes, in fact, even purposely neglecting it. Thus disturbances occurred in the regular course of organic life, and this brought diseases into the world. If, therefore, the gods were directly responsible for the appearance of disease, it was palpably their duty to effect its elimination. Thus it came about that pathology and therapy were exclusively attended to by the gods. But in what light they regarded these medical duties of theirs, and how they performed them, were matters subject to very varying considerations, as expounded by the different religions of antiquity. The Babylonian considered the great god Marduk the expeller of all maladies, whereas Urugal, Namtor, and Nergal were recognized gods of pestilence.

Similar ideas prevailed among the Egyptians. The cat-headed goddess Bubastis was believed to deal out to mothers the blessings of fertility. Ibis showed an especial interest in those human beings who were troubled with disturbances of digestion, and this interest found benevolent expression in the invention of the clyster.

With the Greeks also the gods rendered services to diseased humanity. Thus Apollo invented the art of healing, and if his time permitted he occasionally lent a hand when difficulties beset the entrance into this world of a young mortal. But, as a rule, it was the duty of Aphrodite to attend to such cases, just as, in fact, she was responsible for everything that referred to love, no matter whether it was a question of the esthetic or the pathological part of that passion. Athene was the specialist in ophthalmology, and it seems that she did not fare badly with this occupation. A temple was dedicated to her by Lycurgus, whom, as it appears, she healed of a sympathetic affection of the eyes; and, besides, she won by her ophthalmological activity various ornamental epithets, such, for instance, as ὀφθαλμίτις, etc.

It was quite natural, in view of the exclusively theistic conception which in those times preoccupied the human mind, that the priests were the sole possessors of physico-medical knowledge; and naturally so. For when we consider the theory of life that prevailed at that period, who could have been better qualified to give information to men regarding their own body as well as regarding nature in general, than the priest, the mortal representative of immortal gods? And who better qualified than the priest to invoke the aid of the heavenly powers in all bodily ailments? Thus it was the unavoidable consequence of the theistic theory of life that the priest was the physician as well as the representative of physical knowledge and also the helper and adviser in all mundane exigencies. Whether bodily or psychic troubles afflicted individuals, whether an entire population groaned under heavy chastisements like pestilence, aid and deliverance were always sought in the sanctuary of the gods, from the infallible priest. And the priests were always equal to the occasion; they have always, in a masterly manner, known the art of satisfying the medico-physical needs of their suppliants. For the religions of all civilized peoples—and Christianity by no means occupies an exceptional position in this respect—have always endeavored most strenuously to keep physical as well as medical thought in strictest dependence upon their doctrines and dogmas. To attain this end various ceremonies, customs, and dogmas were relied upon to keep the priests in a position to secure the assistance of the gods for humanity harassed by pain and affliction. These sacred observances were strange, and varied with the various religious systems. According to the primeval cult of Zoroaster, all evils, consequently also all diseases, were derived from the principle of darkness which was embodied in the person of Ahriman, and only the sacerdotal caste of the magicians who sprung from a special Median tribe was able to heal them. But it was by no means easy to become a member of this caste and to acquire the magic powers pertaining to it alone. It was necessary before gaining mastery over the powers of nature to become initiated into the mysteries of Mitra. However, after priestly consecration had once been bestowed, the individual thus honored bore the proud title "Conqueror of Evil," and was able to practise medicine. As the most essential constituent of every medical treatment, the divine word was applied in the form of mysterious exorcisms, sacred hymns, and certain words which were considered specially curative in effect, particularly the word "Ormuzd," the name of the highest god, in whose all-embracing power of healing great confidence was placed.

The Sumerians, the precursors of Babylonico-Assyrian culture, ascribed a considerable and important rôle to dreams. They were considered to bring direct medical advice from the gods, and it became the office of the sacerdotal physician to interpret the dream in such a way as to alleviate the sufferings of the dreamer.

The ancient Greek culture also conceded a conspicuous medical significance to dreams, and even arranged a system of its own, that of the temple sleep, in order always to obtain prophesying dreams from the gods. The patient, after the obligatory offering, was required to remain a night in the temple, and his dream during this night was the medical advice of the divinity in its most direct form. But only the priest was able to interpret a dream obtained in such a manner, and to extract medical efficacy from it. But as it occasionally happened that a too prosaic and phlegmatic patient did not dream at all, the priest was benevolent enough to intercede. He was always promptly favored by the gods with a suggestive dream.

The medical function of the priests had reached a peculiar development during the first centuries of Rome. This was manifest especially in the time of public calamities, such as pestilence, war, etc. When such events reached dimensions which threatened the existence of the republic, attempts were made to gain the favor of the gods by most curious ceremonies. The celestials were simply invited to take part in an opulent banquet. The first divine feast of such a character was celebrated in Rome in the sixth century, B.C., on account of a great epidemic. Apollo, Latona, Diana, Hercules, Mercury, and Neptune were most ceremoniously invited to take part in a religious banquet which lasted for eight days. The images of the gods were placed upon magnificently cushioned couches, and the tables were loaded with dainties. Not only the gods, but the entire population, were invited; every one kept open house, and whoever wished to do so could feast at the richly prepared boards of the wealthy. Even the pronounced enemies of the house were allowed to enter and to enjoy the dainties without fear of hostile remarks; indeed, it was deemed advisable in the interests of public hygiene to unchain the prisoners and to liberate them. But if the gods, in spite of the most opulent entertainments, did not have any consideration, and if pestilence, military disaster, failure of crops, or whatever was the immediate cause of popular anxiety, continued to persist with unabated fury, endeavors were made by theatrical performances to provide as much as possible for the amusement of the gods. Such plays, at first, consisted only in graceful dances, with flute accompaniments, and from these simple beginnings, according to Livy, Book 7, Chapter II., the drama is said to have developed all those variations which characterized the scenic art of antiquity. There can be no doubt that even the stage of modern times is of religio-sanitary origin—a peculiar fact which modern patrons of the theater scarcely ever dream of.

An attempt was eventually made to increase the delight of the gods in such amusements by a number of novel devices. For instance, it was stipulated that the performances instituted to ward off the invasion of Hannibal were to cost 333,333⅓ copper asses. But if, nevertheless, the gods were not sufficiently propitiated by banquets, dances, and playing of the flute, and if they could not be prevailed upon by such pastimes to remove the pestilence or other calamity, a dictator was named who, if possible, on September 13th, drove a nail into the temple of Jupiter to appease divine indignation. It appears that this was a primeval custom of the Etruscans; at least, it is reported by the Roman author, Cincius, that such nails could be seen in the temple of the Etruscan goddess Nortia. This nail therapy was resorted to by the Romans, for instance, during the terrible plague which raged in the fifth century, B.C., and of which the celebrated Furius Camillus died.

Wonderful as all the described procedures seem to us, and closely as they may conform to the modern conception of superstition, at the time they originated they were considered as quite removed from that superstition with which we so closely identify them to-day. For the period which saw the above events was an era of exclusive theism, and for that reason divine sleep, divine feasts, the sacred performances, and all the other peculiar means which were employed to secure medical aid of the gods, were well-established features of religious worship. The stigma of superstition was not set upon them as yet. And this state of things naturally persisted so long as the theistic theory of life stood unchallenged.

This absolute reign of theistic theory dominating human life through the above-described therapeutic ideas was followed by an epoch in which theism was forced to divide its authority with a powerful rival— namely, the physico-mechanical theory of life. The struggle between both these systems was ushered in, for the Hellenic as well as for the Occidental world of civilization, by the appearance of Ionian philosophy. Even in our own day this struggle is still going on in many minds. This much, at least, is certain: that superstition has always been especially active in medicine in areas of civilization where the theistic idea has gained the ascendency.

The deadly struggle between theistic and physico-mechanical theories of life in the realm of medicine has found no place in the experience of Hellenic and Roman antiquity. The change in opinion was rather wrought by a gradual recession from the idea that the gods interfered with the proper course of man's bodily functions. This conviction resulted from a progressive growth of his physico-mechanical knowledge, and became established at least as far as the thoughts and the opinions of the physicians were concerned. That the other classes, in particular the representatives of religion, did not so peaceably acquiesce in this mechanical conception of life we shall soon explain in Chapter III. It was different, however, with the art of healing itself. Even the Corpus Hippocraticum reveals to us a medicine which had been purified from all theistic admixtures, and from the publication of this work (i.e., from about the fifth century, B.C., up to the overthrow of the ancient period—i.e., until about the fifth or sixth century, A.D.) no further attempt to refer the cause of disease and the treatment of disease to the gods of the ancient heavens is noticed in medical works. On the contrary, that great efforts were made to look for the nature of disease in the mechanical conditions of the body is proven by a number of the most various medical doctrines. The extensive work of Galen, that antique canon of medicine, which dates back to the second century, A.D., disavows all theism and all theurgy, and relies solely upon physico-mechanical methods: observation, experiment, dissection. Antique religion and antique medicine had effected a reconciliation— a reconciliation, however, in which neither party was to acknowledge a complete defeat; but the result was an amicable settlement, in which their just dues were given both to the theistic and to the physico-mechanical theories of life. The point of agreement upon which this settlement, or, to express it better, compromise, was made was teleology.

By teleology we understand the conception that all earthly existence is created by a supreme power in accordance with a preconceived plan, and that, accordingly, all organic life, in form and action, is most perfectly adapted to the task prescribed for it by this power. This conception was absolutely indispensable to antique medicine; for it allowed the adherents of the theistic theory without hesitation to consider man as a product of the creator, which was distinguished in all directions and which bore witness of the wisdom of God, a position which precluded the assumption, which was impossible according to the antecedent medical observations, that disease came from God. For it seemed quite plausible, according to the physico-mechanical theory of life, that disease might be a product of a number of adverse, purely earthly conditions, an assumption not involving the slightest doubt of the wisdom and creative power of the gods. This teleological doctrine, which runs like a red thread through all ancient philosophy, becomes conspicuously prominent in Galen. Every section of the powerful work of Galen—anatomy, as well as physiology, pathology, and therapy—bear witness to the most confident teleological conception, a conception which in the end culminates in the verdict ("Use of the Parts," Book 11, Chapter XIV.): "The creator of nature has disclosed his benevolence by wise care for all his creatures, in that he has bestowed upon each one what is truly of service to it."

This teleological idea of all earthly becoming, being, and passing away was henceforth destined to be a permanent factor in human speculation. Christianity received it as a possession from antique civilization, and only the philosophy and natural science of modern times have been able to threaten its permanence. Biology, as of modern creation, teaches us that all natural phenomena owe their existence to natural causes, that the natural world is subject to natural laws. And, accordingly, teleology, as we encounter it in the works of the heathen Galen and in the writings of the Christian Church Fathers, has turned out to be superstition, which, however, must by no means be classed with the vagaries of mere medico-physical superstition. In coming to this decision, however, we must beware of rash generalization. In this connection we refer only to that kind of teleology which dominated the world previous to the teachings of Descartes and Spinoza, and previous to the advent of modern natural science, with its biological methods. Whether, after all, a theory of life might be possible which, while avoiding the reproach of superstition, might be traced to teleological prepossessions, is a question we can not here discuss. It is admittedly true that the deeper we penetrate into the secrets of nature the more energetically the existence of a marvelous, intelligent will manifests itself as permeating all domains of nature. However, if this fact is not denied on principle, as modern materialism denies it, and proper allowance is made for it, a rehabilitation of teleology as a necessary factor of our theory of life would be the logical consequence. Of course, this teleology would bear a stamp entirely different from that of antiquity and of the middle ages, which is recognized to be superstition. It should not pretend to include the consideration of the entire organic world, but confine its conclusions to the last links in the chain of experience and argument which science has forged from natural phenomena. Now this could be accomplished, in our opinion, even without apprehension of interfering with the indispensable requirements of modern naturalists: "The terrestrial world in its forms and processes is governed solely by terrestrial laws." What the appearance of such a teleology should be is expressed by William Hartpole Lecky in the following:

"This conception, which exhibits the universe rather as an organism than a mechanism, and regards the complexities and adaptations it displays rather as the results of gradual development from within than of an interference from without, is so novel, and at first sight so startling, that many are now shrinking from it in alarm, under the impression that it destroys the argument from design, and almost amounts to the negation of a Supreme Intelligence. But there can, I think, be little doubt that such fears are, for the most part, unfounded. That matter is governed by mind, that the contrivances and elaborations of the universe are the products of intelligence, are propositions which are quite unshaken, whether we regard these contrivances as the result of a single momentary exercise of will, or of a slow, consistent, and regulated evolution. The proofs of a pervading and developing intelligence, and the proofs of a coordinating and combining intelligence, are both untouched, nor can any conceivable progress of science in this direction destroy them. If the famous suggestion, that all animal and vegetable life results from a single vital germ, and that all the different animals and plants now existent were developed by a natural process of evolution from that germ, were a demonstrated truth, we should still be able to point to the evidence of intelligence displayed in the measured and progressive development, in those exquisite forms so different from what blind chance could produce, and in the manifest adaptation of surrounding circumstances to the living creature, and of the living creature to surrounding circumstances. The argument from design would indeed be changed; it would require to be stated in a new form, but it would be fully as cogent as before. Indeed, it is, perhaps, not too much to say that the more fully this conception of universal evolution is grasped, the more firmly a scientific doctrine of Providence will be established, and the stronger will be the presumption of a future progress."[1]

In such a manner, despite the fact that in teleology the point of agreement between theistic and physico-mechanical medical thought has been now found, theism, in the course of the history of our science, continually attempted new attacks upon the physical tendency in medicine; and with each assault superstition in medicine, as well as in the natural sciences, was most palpably exposed.

After having satisfied ourselves in this second chapter regarding theism and its attitude with reference to the physico-mechanical theory of life, we shall now enter upon the consideration of the various forms of medical superstition, and it is our intention, as stated in the first chapter, so to arrange the enormous material at hand as to discuss medical superstition according to the sources from which it has sprung. We shall begin by pointing out the intimate relations which have prevailed between the teachings of religion and superstition.

---

[1] "History of the Rise and Influence of the Spirit of Rationalism in Europe," Vol. I., Chapter III., pages 294-295. Compare also Magnus, "Medicine and Religion," page 24, sqq.

III

RELIGION THE SUPPORT OF MEDICAL SUPERSTITION

RELIGION undoubtedly plays the most conspicuous part in the history of medical superstition. Religious teaching, of whatever character, has fostered medical superstition more than any other factor of civilization. Not only has religion called forth and nourished medical superstition, but it has also defended it with all the influence at its disposal. Indeed, it has not infrequently happened that those who were reluctant to believe in the blessings of a medical theory ridiculously perverted by religion were exposed to persecution by fire and sword. And this not only from one or other religious denomination, for all religious believers, without exception, had proved to be the most assiduous promotors of medical superstition; so that we are probably not wrong in designating priesthoods in general, whatever their creed, as the most prominent embodiment of medical superstition during certain periods of the world's history. But the details will be learned from the following paragraphs:

§ 1. **Priesthood the Support of Medical Superstition.**—The principal reason for a not quite reputable activity in the chosen representative of a deity is probably the fact that, with the appearance of a physico-mechanical contemplation of the world, the theistic theory of life, which until then had exclusive sway, was forced into a pitched battle with a newly formulated definition of nature. This struggle was carried on principally by the priesthood, who, as a matter of fact, had most to lose from the ascendency of a new theory of life which only reckoned with natural factors. They indeed had been the means, until then, of procuring for the people the assistance of the gods in all bodily ailments, as they had been the exclusive depositories of physical knowledge. And it could scarcely be expected that the priesthood would at once willingly relinquish the extensive supremacy hitherto exercised by it as the oracle of divine guidance in all medico-physical questions; for humanity has always considered the possession of authority much more delightful than submission, and the ruler has always objected most energetically to any attempt which disputes his rule. This was precisely what was done by priests of all creeds when the mechanico-physical theory of life began to supersede the obsolete dreams of theistic medicine. Fair-minded persons will surely allow that such action was natural. But they can not approve of the methods resorted to, unless they belong to those who feel bound always to discern nothing but what is sacred in every action of a servant of heaven.

In order to wage war most effectively against the physico-mechanical theory of life, the priesthood at once claimed for themselves the power of completely controlling nature. They made the people believe that the celestials had bestowed upon them the faculty of dominating nature in the interests of the sick, and that all powers of the universe, the obvious ones as well as those mysteriously hidden in the depths of nature, were obedient to sacerdotal suggestions. The servant of heaven professed that he could regulate the eternal processes of matter, with its becoming, being, and passing away, quite as irresistibly as his eye was able to survey the course of time in the past, present, and future.

Equipped with these extensive powers, a priest necessarily appeared to the people not only as physician, but also as a miraculous being crowned with the halo of the supernatural. And this was the rôle he actually played in many ancient religions. With the peoples of Italy the priest appeared—at a period, indeed, which was previous to the beginning of Rome—as physician, prophet, interpreter of dreams, raiser of tempests, etc. He held exactly the same offices among the Celtic tribes in Gaul and Britain. His position was the same in the Oriental world, and by the Medians and the Persians especially were priests considered to be persons endowed with supernatural powers. We may notice that members of a certain Median tribe formed the sacerdotal caste, and bore the name of "Magi." However, this name, which originally was confined to the priestly order, obtained, in the course of time, a distinctly secular meaning. Very soon many cunning fellows arrived at the conclusion that the trade of a sacerdotal physician and conjurer might bring a profitable livelihood to its professor, even if this professor were not a priest but a layman. Thus there arose a special profession of sorcerers, miracle workers, and medicine-men, who protested with solemn emphasis that they were able to cure all physical as well as psychical ailments of their fellow men as thoroughly as the priests had done. But in order to bestow the required consecration upon this art, these gentlemen usurped the venerable name of the above-mentioned Median sacerdotal caste and called themselves "Magi." Thus it happened that the name "Magus" (magician), which originally served to designate a distinct sacerdotal caste, deteriorated into a designation of charlatans and swindlers. This could never have occurred unless the priests had prostituted their sublime profession and degraded it to various kinds of discreditable medico-physical deceptions. This alone is why priesthood is responsible for the rise of the magicians, of these worthless fakirs. But if Pliny (Book 30, Chapter I., § 2) attempts to rank magic as an offshoot of medicine, he is justified in doing so only in so far as the priest, during the theistic period, was also the physician, as is well known. Only from this point of view is it possible to trace a genetic relation between medicine and magic. But medicine in itself has not taken the slightest part in the promotion of magic and the success of its unsavory reputation. Indeed, our science has suffered too much through the practise of magic to burden itself with the paternity of this disreputable child of civilization.

It appears that the name of the Celtic priests ("druids") had become subject to the same abuse as the name of the Median priests of sacerdotal caste. Thus we learn of female fortune-tellers of the third century, A.D., who call themselves "druidesses." But it seems that this application of the word "druid" has remained a local one and strictly limited, whereas the expression "magician," quite generally employed, became, in the course of time, the designation of charlatans and medical impostors. For these swindlers, who carried on medico-physical hocuspocus, and who claimed to exercise supernatural powers, were called "magicians" during the entire period of classic antiquity, and we find the same use of the word in the middle ages, and sometimes also in more modern times.

But this profession of magician, which sprang from priesthood, has largely promoted superstition in medicine, and was particularly instrumental in bringing it into extraordinary repute. It is our intention to concern ourselves a little more minutely with magicians and magic.

§2. **The Spread of the Word "Magic."**—How and when magic was transplanted from its Oriental home to the Occident can not be determined with certainty; for the Greeks, as well as all antique peoples, probably all nations, had a belief in ghosts and demons, in fortune-telling, and in sorcery. But it appears, nevertheless, that the ancient civilized peoples of the Orient, and particularly the Persians, cultivated the magic arts with especial devotion, and it is more than probable that it was from the East that theprevailing cult of magic had been imported into the West. Pliny, for one, tells us (Book 30, Chapter I., § 8) that magic was brought to Europe by a certain Osthanes, who accompanied King Xerxes on his military expedition against Greece. This man Osthanes, as Pliny reports further, is said to have disseminated the seeds of this supernatural art (*velut semina artis portentosæ insparsit*) wherever he went, and with such success that the Hellenic peoples were actually mad after it, and prominent men traveled through parts of the Orient, there to acquire personally and thoroughly these magic arts, thus, as was the case with Pythagoras, Empedocles, Democritus, and Plato. In fact, it is said of Democritus that he opened the tomb of a celebrated magician—Dardanus of Phœnicia—that he might restore to publicity the mysterious writings of the latter. It appears, moreover, that Alexander the Great entertained an implicit belief in magic—at least, Pliny reports that during his wars he was always accompanied by a celebrated magician.

Magic arts were likewise in favor among the Romans. Even Nero attempted to master the secrets of magic, altho unsuccessfully (Pliny, Book 30, Chapter II., § 5). A particular impetus was given to magic toward the end of the last century before Christ and during the first century of the Christian era, when the rise of many fantastic philosophical systems greatly promoted and supported the belief in the supernatural powers of magic. Subsequently, in the middle ages, magic experienced an accepted and systematic development. These conditions, however, will be more explicitly referred to later on.

The treatment of the sick through supernatural agencies assumed quite astonishing dimensions under the Roman emperors. The belief in magicians was so generally disseminated that even the emperors themselves and the imperial authorities were almost completely devoted to it. Thus, for instance, the emperor Hadrian (117-138, A.D.) caused himself to be treated by physicians who claimed miraculous powers, and he is said to have written a book on theurgy. In fact, Suidas (62 Julianus) reports that Hadrian, on account of a severe outbreak of pestilence in Rome, sent for the son of the Chaldean, Julian, who, simply by the power of his miracles, arrested the progress of the disease. Under Antoninus Pius official proclamations were made in the forum, directing the attention of the people to the importance of magicians (Philostratus, 43), and the emperor Marcus Aurelius even relates that, when in Caieta, the gods in a dream prescribed a remedy for the hemorrhagic cough and vertigo from which he was suffering ("Marcus Aurelius," Chapter I., § 17, page 11).

But it appears that the magicians finally went too far with their tricks, and endangered human life by their treatment; so that several emperors decided upon adopting more rigorous measures against their knaveries. The emperor Septimius Severus (193-211), altho himself originally devoted to magic, prohibited, when on a visit in Egypt, all books which taught curious arts (Aelius Spartianus, "Hadrianus," Chapter XV., § 5, page 146). Later the emperor Diocletian took energetic steps toward abating the mischief done by magical treatment of the sick, and the magicians were permitted to carry on such arts only so far as would not be detrimental to the health of the people. However, this order did not check the magicians any more than it benefited those who were still tortured and brought to the point of death by magic quackery. Neither did medical science derive any advantage whatever from this well-meant but completely abortive effort of the emperor, for the magic physicians persisted in carrying on their hocuspocus, and unconcernedly debased the pharmacopœia by the introduction of nonsensical and loathsome substances. Let us examine more in detail this department of medical practise among the magicians.

§ 3. **The Medical Practise of the Magicians.**— The magicians adopted various modes of procedure in the treatment of the sick: they either attempted, as do our modern quacks, to create the impression, by administering medicine, that they were actually able to direct the treatment of the ailing in a rational manner, or they restricted themselves to various kinds of magical observances.

The drug therapy of the magicians actually utilized everything under the sun as a remedy. The more out of the way and the less suitable for a remedy a substance seemed to be, the more likely it was to be chosen by the magician intent upon healing. For it was always the main object of these practising quacks to make their treatment as sensational as possible. In this they succeeded best by employing the most extraordinary substances as remedies. Thus they made use of gold, silver, precious stones and pearls, just because these, owing to their value, were held in great esteem, and their medical application, therefore, was bound to create a sensation. But the most loathsome substances were quite as readily employed, for here, too, the most general attention was bound to be attracted by their application. Human feces, urine, and menstrual blood were introduced into the materia medica in such a manner. The awe with which parts of corpses usually inspired the non-medical part of the public was relied upon by the magicians to advertise their cures. Thus these quacks administered powders of human bones to the ailing.

But inasmuch as what is conspicuous and unusual has always enjoyed an especial esteem with humanity, the incredible remedies of the magicians naturally found everywhere an abundance of believers; and as particularly the most nonsensical theory is most tenacious of life, provided it has been presented in apparent combination with the miraculous, the medical armamentarium rapidly took on a very peculiar aspect. Until the present more modern times medicine was condemned to the encumbrance of this rubbish, this list of odd and loathsome remedies, whose admission to the pharmacopœia was only due to the whim of a human mind that constantly hankers after the extraordinary and the miraculous.

Finally the magic observances to which the magicians resorted in the treatment of the sick, have shown a remarkable vitality, for they are in vogue even in modern times, and many sections of our people even to-day swear unconditionally by the curative efficacy of various agencies which demonstratively have been derived from the medicine of the magicians. But now such agencies are no longer ascribed to magic or sorcery, but they are called "cures by means of sympathy." And as many modern people believe that various incomprehensible mystic performances cause certain mysterious powers, otherwise absolutely unknown, to exert a curative influence upon certain diseases, so did the ancients believe exactly the same. This was the origin of exorcism as a remedy for disease. Exorcism played a conspicuous part in the middle ages as a means of stopping hemorrhages, and even in these modern times, as is well-known, this method of cure finds many adherents.

This magic treatment was believed to be especially efficacious if the exorcisms had been written or engraved upon paper, gold, precious stones, etc., in which case they were suspended around the neck of the patient. Countless talismans (from the Arabic *tilsam*, magic image) and amulets (from the Arabic*hamalet*, trinket) were thus manufactured, and even to our own time there are survivals of this medical superstition. Altho these mystic observances are performed in various ways, and their modifications are practically innumerable, yet certain radical resemblances are continually appearing among the magic rites of the most diverse races, and some of these practises have even persisted up to the present time. Thus the rope of the hung criminal plays a conspicuous part in antique magic as well as in modern sympathy treatment; the same importance is attributed to shooting-stars, to the moon, to crossroads, to certain numerals, such as 3, 7, 9, etc. It is a highly interesting fact that such conceptions, as remarkable for their therapeutical associations as for their crass superstition, are possessed of a vitality which persists for centuries. Peoples, religions, philosophical systems, political revolutions have risen and vanished, but the belief in the curative action of the rope of a hung criminal or the therapeutic significance of the crossroad has survived. The mystic influence which is exerted by the numerals 3, 7, 9, and still more so by the dreadful 13, upon the life and health of man, haunts the minds of the multitude in this century of physical enlightenment exactly as it did in remote antiquity. But we can not here enter into the reason for these interesting facts, and we must refer those who desire more detailed information on this subject to the voluminous literature of superstition.

Furthermore, the belief in magic cures was not more prevalent among the ancient professors of medicine than among the laity, and even the most prominent practitioners were not able to emancipate themselves from this belief. Galen, for instance, who, as is well-known, mastered the entire literature of antique medicine as none before or after him has ever done, openly avows his belief in the efficacy of magic cures, and, what is more remarkable, Galen in this respect has changed from a Saul to a Paul. He ruefully recalled, later, the condemnatory decree which he had originally promulgated regarding the magic treatment of the sick. Let us call to mind how he expresses himself in his essay on medical treatment in Homer: "Many, as I have done for a long time, believe that conjurations resemble the fairy tales of old women. But gradually, and from the observation of obvious facts, I have come to the conclusion that power is exercised by them; for I have learned to know their advantages in stings of scorpions, and also in bones which became lodged in the throat, and which were at once coughed up as a result of conjuration. Many remedies are excellent in every respect, and magic formulæ answer their purpose" ("Alexander of Tralles," Book 11, Chapter I., Vol. II., page 477). One of the most prominent post-Galenian physicians also, Alexander of Tralles, openly avows, with reference to this utterance of Galen, that he himself is a believer in magic cures, and he says: "If the great Galen, as well as many other physicians of ancient times, bear witness to this fact (the efficacy of magic treatment of the sick), why shall we not impart to you what we have learned from our own experience and what we have heard from trustworthy friends?" ("Alexander of Tralles," ibid.). Accordingly, his Βιβλία Ἰατρικά was filled with enumerations of the most various magical cures. But, now, if the classics of antique medicine have proven themselves to be so friendly to the medical science of magicians, what was the condition of the mind, then, of the average physician of ancient times? Is it astonishing if young and old, high and low, without distinction, were blind adherents of magical medicine? Thus medical literature of the last century,B.C., and especially that of the centuries from the Christian era until late in the middle ages, was an actual treasury of conjuration and other mummeries. This description applies specifically to the "Materia Medica" of Quintus Serenus Samonicus, written in hexameters. It is true, the magical sequel to this book entailed painful consequences on the writer, for the emperor Caracalla had the poor author executed (Ael. Spartian., "Caracalla," Chapter IV., § 4) merely, as it is reported, because he dared to advise in his works as a remedy against intermittent fever the wearing of amulets, a medical expedient which had been prohibited by the emperor himself.

The work of Sextus Placitus Papyriensis, who lived in the fourth century, which treats of remedies derived from the animal kingdom, teems with magic nonsense.

But an actually inexhaustible stock of medical conjurations was contained in the work of a layman, Marcellus Empiricus. This gentleman, who had been foreign minister under the emperors Theodosius the first and the second, had written a thick folio volume on medicaments. This literary performance, which, according to our ideas, appears to be very odd for a minister of state, was by no means remarkable in the fifth century, for the study of medical subjects was, so to say, fashionable among the laity of that period; in fact, even prelates and bishops did not think it beneath their dignity to busy themselves with various medical questions and to write medico-physical books. Thus the laurels of medical renown haunted our good Marcellus and would not let him sleep, so that he abridged his hours of official duty to such an extent that he was able to compile a Materia Medica of thirty-six apparently never-ending chapters. But if the statesmanship of Marcellus was on a par with his medical book-making, the two Theodosii could not have missed the time their cabinet minister stole from them, for his medical scribbling is an utterly worthless compilation. Not only did Marcellus copy from medical authors of the most discordant opinion, but he particularly busied himself in collecting indiscriminately all the magical nonsense of the ancient times; in fact, it seems that he was very eager to obtain all this magical rigmarole direct from the mouth of the people, for he says that he collected his remedies "*ab agrestibus et plebeiis.*" Accordingly his book is as worthless and insipid to the physician as it is valuable to the historian, especially the historian of civilization. Here are a few examples of this medicine of the magicians:

Remedy against warts and corns (Pliny, Book 28, Chapter IV., § 12, page 268): "Lie on your back along a boundary line on the twentieth day of the moon, and extend the hands over the head. With whatever thing you grasp when so doing, rub the warts, and they will disappear immediately."

"Whoever, when he sees a shooting-star, soon afterward pours a little vinegar upon the hinge of a door, is sure to be rid of his corns."

Remedy against headache (Pliny, ibid.): "Tie the rope of a hung criminal around the forehead."

Remedy against bellyache (Priscian, physician of the fourth century, Book 1, Chapter XIV., and Sprengel, Vol. II., page 248): "If any one suffer from colicky pains he may sit down on a chair and say to himself: '*Per te diacholon, diacholon, diacholon.*'"

"A person who has an attack of colic may take the feces of a wolf, which, if possible, should contain small particles of bone, enclose them in a small tube, and wear this amulet on the right arm, thigh, or hip."—*Alexander of Tralles*, Book 8, Chapter II., page 374.

"Take the heart from the living lark and wear it as an amulet at the left thigh."—*Alexander of Tralles, ibid.*

Remedy against epilepsy (advised by the physician, Moschion Diorthotes. "Alexander of Tralles," Book 1, Chapter XV., page 570): "The forehead of an ass is tied to the skin of the patient and worn."

"Gather iris, peonies, and nightshade when the moon is on the wane, pack them into linen and wear as an amulet." Advised by the magician Osthanes.—*Alexander of Tralles*, Book 1, Chapter XV., page 566.

"Take a nail from a cross and suspend it from an arm of the patient." Given by a physician of the second century, A.D., by the name of Archigenes.—*Alexander of Tralles*, Book 1, Chapter XV., page 566.

"Wear on the finger a jasper of bluish-gray luster."—Advised by *Dioscorides*, Book 5, 159.

Remedy against podagra [gout] ("Alexander of Tralles," Book 12, page 582): "Take a gold leaf and write upon it when the moon is on the wane: mei, threu, mor, for, teux, za, zon, the, lu, chri, ge, ze, on. As the sun becomes firm in this name and daily renews itself, so does this formation also make firm as conditions were previously. Quickly, quickly, rapidly, rapidly. For behold! I call the great name in which becomes firm again what was destined to die: Jas, azyf, zyon, threux, dain, chook. Make this formation firm as it has been, quickly, quickly, rapidly, rapidly. This document must be covered with the tendon of a crane, enclosed in a capsule, and worn by the patient at his heel."

Remedy against diseases of the eye (advised by Sextus Placitus Papyriensis. Magnus, "Ophthalmology of the Ancients," page 597): "If the right eye becomes afflicted with glaucoma, rub it with the right eye of the wolf, and, similarly, the left eye with the left eye of the wolf."

In photophobia (fear of light) "Wear as an amulet an eye which was taken from a live crab."—*Quintus Serenus Samonicus.* Magnus, "Ophthalmology of the Ancients," page 595.

With pains of the eye the patient must, with a copper needle, put out the eyes of a green lizard caught on a Jupiter day, during a moon that is on the wane, in the month of September. The eyes must be worn in a golden capsule, as an amulet around the neck (*Marcellus Empiricus.* Magnus, "Ophthalmology of the Ancients," page 602.)

The above illustrations are surely sufficient to give the reader an idea of the medicine of the magicians. At the same time they show the great similarity which exists between these ancient magic cures and the sympathetic cures of our people at the present day.

§ 4. **Ancient Medicine and Magic.**—But how is it possible that the ancient physicians, and even the most enlightened minds among them, should not only have tolerated such a crass medical superstition as the above examples have shown us, but should even have incorporated them in their works? Incomprehensible, however, as this fact may appear to the modern practitioner, it becomes conceivable if the condition of antique medicine and of the medical profession of ancient times is considered.

In the first place, ancient medical science adopted an entirely different mode of diagnostico-theoretical method than that employed by professors of medicine in modern times. Ancient natural science (compare also Chapter V. of this work), as well as ancient medicine, obtained their scientific views exclusively by deduction—i.e., they deduced individual results from general presumptions, or, rather, they construed, by reason of some general presumption, the physico-medical consequences which were to follow from such a general supposition. If this attempt to obtain an insight into physical processes is extremely hazardous, it becomes still more precarious when the manner and means in which these general presumptions were arrived at were primarily of an entirely hypothetical nature. It is true, no fundamental objection can be raised to this method, as even modern natural science and medicine, despite the fact that their methods of investigation in a diagnostico-theoretical respect scarcely admit of material objections, can not do without hypothesis. But hypothesis is not always mere hypothesis. It is well known that there are hypotheses which, even in the minds of the most conscientious investigators, are not inferior to that knowledge which is obtained by experiment and observation, whereas other hypotheses again present the distinct stamp of insufficiency and makeshift. The trustworthiness and the heuristic value of an hypothesis depend upon the quality of the diagnostico-theoretical process by means of which it was obtained. If this process has been such as physical investigation is bound to insist upon, the hypothesis thus arrived at is fully justified to supply the still absent data with regard to the phenomena in question. This, however, can be accomplished by hypothesis only when the latter is not set forth until it plainly appears that, in spite of a conscientious and orderly arrangement of observation after observation, of experiment upon experiment, without the admission of logical loopholes, full data in regard to the nature of the phenomena is not forthcoming. In such a case we may consider as actually proven by hypothesis what observation and systematic experiment, continuous and logical, were intended to prove, and failed. However, this inductive hypothesis is alone entitled to be considered in medicine. Naturally, such an inductive hypothesis was not thought of by the ancients, as the inductive method of investigation was generally quite unknown to them. The process by which ancient medicine usually attempted to find its hypothesis was by an argument from analogy. Each and every point of resemblance, however superficial, between two phenomena was considered sufficient by the ancient naturalists to warrant the assumption that analogous phenomena in the most various domains were most certainly proven to possess similar points of resemblance. And upon the basis of such an insecure method of deduction—which, moreover, was selected entirely at the option of the observer—the ancient investigator erected the boldest hypotheses. Thus, for instance, the atomic theory of Leucippus and

Democritus is an hypothesis which rests upon the basis of a conclusion from analogy. The motes which appear in the rays of the sun led these two ancient investigators to the conception that, like the particles of dust sporting in the air, the primary component parts of everything that exists in the entire universe consisted of similar particles.[2]

It appears that Epicurus arrived at his theory of light (according to which, as is well known, images of things were brought to the senses by delicate but absolutely objective small pictures which were detached from the surface of things in a continuous current) by the fact that many animals—for instance, snakes—shed their skins. The theory of humoral pathology, one of the most important advances in medical science, was based on a conclusion from analogy and arrived at by the deductive method.

The diagnostico-theoretical lines in which antique medicine moved were bound—and this is the point of importance in this case—to exert a determining influence upon medical criticism. For medico-physical criticism can only appear in closest connection with the prevailing condition of the respective sciences, being really nothing else but a precipitate from them. Thus the ancient physicians were compelled to take an entirely different position toward magical medicine than we moderns, educated in the school of inductive methods, have always taken. The probable and similar, the supposable and possible, in which deductive medicine found its data,

---

[2] Lucretius, Book 2, Verse 113, sqq.

working on the lines of argument from analogy, were necessarily bound to find expression also in the character of medical critique, and it was impossible, therefore, for the ancient physician to detect anything absurd or contrary to experience in hypotheses which the practitioner of to-day at once brands as nonsensical and superstitious.

We are not in the least justified, therefore, in speaking disparagingly of Galen and Alexander of Tralles because they believed in magical medicine and applied it in their practise. As no human being can jump out of his skin, so is he unable to get beyond the intellectual advancement of his time. As the ancient physicians were also unable to do this, accordingly they were believers in the magical medicine.

But there is still a second point which explains the remarkable position taken by ancient physicians in relation to magical medicine—namely, the fact that the conception of miracle and magic were essentially different in the ancient world from what they are at present. The belief in the interference of spirits and supernatural beings in terrestrial matters, and the manifestations of their influence exerted in manifold ways—sometimes for good, sometimes for evil—had been widely disseminated from the earliest times, and we encounter them in all periods of classic antiquity. This belief in demons had become incorporated in the systems of many leading philosophers of antiquity. Now if the world were filled with demons the natural consequence was that their activity would manifest itself in various ways. It was necessary, therefore, that man should always be prepared to experience manifestations which more or less violated the customary order of terrestrial happenings, and for this reason nothing that could be styled a miracle really existed for him. A miracle could not be conceived in its full modern sense until it was realized that the course of all natural phenomena was nothing but the expression of eternal and changeless laws. However, it was not until comparatively late that this conception became generally disseminated; thus, for instance, it was considered as self-evident, even in the latest periods of the middle ages and during the first beginnings of modern times, that divine influence could always, and actually did always, cause an alteration in the course of the functions of the body. In fact, there is an amazingly large number of people even in our time who believe this, and for whom, therefore, the conception of miracles, especially of miraculous healing, is to-day on about the same level as that on which it stood in the time of Galen and Alexander of Tralles.

Thus we must admit that the ancient physicians were by no means below the standard of civilization and culture attained during their period if they believed in the possibility of extraordinary cures effected by means extraneous and unscientific in their treatment of the sick, and, accordingly, they supported suchmethods. However, this belief in miraculous medicines on the part of the ancient physician was always restricted to certain limits. It is true, the conception was always adhered to that this or that magical agency, or this or that magical action, might exert an influence upon the disease; but such a belief never led them to omit any strictly medical measures of a surgical or gynecological nature. On the contrary, the intelligent physicians of antiquity firmly insisted that the actions of the surgeon and of the gynecologist were not to be hampered by any metaphysical considerations; thus, for instance, Soranus demanded most energetically that the midwife should be "ἀδεισιδαίμων" (without fear of any demon)—i.e., she was not to be superstitious, but free from any imputation which would render her curative interposition objectionable.

The profession of the magicians, due to the persecutions to which they became subject under the Christian emperors Valens, Valentinian, and Theodosius, became considerably less prominent during the predominance of Christianity, but the ideas upon which it had been erected in ancient times still survived; in fact, these ideas were even to a certain extent systematically elaborated during the middle ages, and at this time a distinction was made between higher and lower, or white and black, magic. The white magic busied itself with good spirits, the black magic with the bad ones. Magicians, therefore, who operated by the aid of the devil, and even in medicine called in the assistance of the devil, were called "necromancers." For the first time magic became amalgamated with certain philosophical speculations and also with Christian-dogmatic constituents. The methods adopted by magic medicine under these conditions are so peculiar and are so close to the boundary lines between philosophy and religion that we are really not quite certain whether to relegate it to the domain of one or of the other. But as the fundamental parts of these methods were actually supplied by philosophy, we propose to defer this discussion for the present, and to take up here another form of medical superstition which was derived exclusively from religion—namely, "sleep in the temple."

§ 5. **Sleep in the Temple.**—One of the generally practised methods of medical science during the period of Hellenic civilization which was still fully under the influence of theism—i.e., for at least two or three centuries before the Hippocratic era—was what was known as "temple sleep." In fact, this method must be considered a sign of a faith distinctly deep and sincere, a faith naive and childlike indeed; but as a sign of such a faith this method is actually pathetic. No taint of superstition could be found in it at the early period referred to. It was still the pure and unadulterated expression of the generally prevailing conception that human art is to no purpose in any case of disease, and aid must be found with the gods—with those gods who regulate and personally execute all terrestrial phenomena down to the minutest details. Temple sleep was not degraded into superstition until medicine had come to the conclusion that the phenomena of disease were not evidence of an interference by supernatural power in the functions of the body, but disturbances of the function of the body caused exclusively by natural causes. In accordance with this view, which first found its fullest and clearest exposition in the *corpus hippocraticum*, it would seem absolutely necessary for temple sleep to lose all recognition from the art of healing. However, this not being the case, it was bound to deteriorate into an act of superstitious mummery, and the principal blame for this sad decadence is to be laid primarily upon the priests. It was their duty especially to lead into the path of truth the patients who persisted in crowding into the temples in the spirit of naive and childlike piety. They sealed their own condemnation as fosterers of superstition when they failed to do this duty, and endeavored rather, by every means in their power, to confirm the multitude in their ancient belief that the gods were practising medicine. Non-Christian as well as Christian priests played this rôle for many centuries with equal ability and equal perseverance, as will be seen from the following brief history of temple sleep.

The belief in the efficacy of temple sleep had already been thoroughly shaken during the time of the great Hippocrates; therefore, in the sixth century, B.C., the laughing philosopher of Hellenism, Aristophanes, the satirical contemporary of Hippocrates, in Act II., verses 654 to 750, of his comedyΠλοῦτος, severely criticizes the manner and method in which temple sleep was employed. Let us listen to the words in which the poet describes what happened in the temple during the observance of this rite.

The god Æsculapius, accompanied by his daughter Panakeia, appears in the temple to examine in person the patients gathered there. The first one he meets is a poor wretch, Neokleides, who, being blear-eyed, expects cure from the god. The medically skilled Æsculapius smears upon the inverted lids of this patient a salve which causes such pain that the poor fellow will probably never seek his help again. The second patient met by the god is the blind god, Πλοῦτος (i.e., Wealth Personified). Here the conduct of Æsculapius is entirely different from that which he adopted when treating poor Neokleides. Now he carefully strokes the head of the patient, then produces a linen cloth and carefully touches the lids with it. He then calls his daughter Panakeia, who winds a red cloth round the head of blind Wealth. Now Æsculapius whistles, and two mighty serpents appear, glide under the purple cloth, and lick the eyes of the patient. Shortly afterward the god regains his sight.

This passage is a cutting satire on practises which undoubtedly prevailed in the Greek temples as early as the sixth century, B.C. But, nevertheless, it took a long time before the patients lost their belief in the miraculous efficacy of temple sleep, and the priesthood continually strove to revive, by the mysterious stories of various kinds they recounted to doubters, the belief in temple sleep. The sixth of the marble votive tablets which were found in the temple of Æsculapius at Epidaurus shows the kind of miraculous reports invented by the priests. The latter were in the habit of inscribing upon these tablets reports of cures that had occurred in their sanctuary, for the benefit of the visitors of the temple and for the still greater benefit of the medical historians; but it is quite probable that the priesthood, intent upon curing, were encouraged in their medico-literary attempts only by the silent hope of creating an abundant supply of patients by such miraculous reports. The above tablet, No. 6—which probably dates from the third century, B.C.—tells us that a blind man by the name of Hermon, a native of Thasos, had recovered his sight by sleeping in the Epidaurean temple of Æsculapius. However, it appears that this man Hermon had been a miserable wretch, for he disappeared without having expressed his thanks in hard cash. Naturally such ingratitude provoked the god, and summarily he blinded the thankless individual again. It required a second temple sleep before the god condescended to become helpful once more. But our tablet does not mention anything about the amount of the remuneration paid by our friend Hermon who had been twice cured of blindness; neither is this at all necessary. The miraculous tablet, even without stating the price, doubtless made sufficient impression upon the minds even of the most parsimonious of future patients.

Altho, therefore, the more enlightened among the Greeks recognized, as early as in the sixth century, B.C., the futility of temple sleep as a means of healing, the ancient world never relinquished it entirely. We encounter it again in the later periods of antiquity. Thus, for instance, Suetonius and other ancient authors tell us that two patients, one blind, the other lame, one day approached the emperor Vespasian, who happened to be in Alexandria, asking him to spit into the eyes of the one and to stroke the paralyzed limbs of the other; for they had been notified in temple sleep that they would be restored to health if only the emperor would deign to perform the above-mentioned manipulations. But Vespasian was an enlightened ruler who, in spite of his imperial dignity, did not have much confidence in the medical qualities of his saliva and of his hands, and accordingly unceremoniously dismissed both supplicants. This caused great terror among the priests of Serapis and among the courtiers, for obviously they had interpreted this affair solely as intended *in majorem Vespasiani gloriam*. The emperor was importuned, therefore, kindly to aid the unfortunate, but he persisted in his refusal. Probably he was right in fearing the loss of his prestige should the imperial medical powers prove unequal to the task of curing disease. Not until the priests solemnly vouched for the truthfulness of the dream-sending god Serapis, and declared a failure of the imperial cure to be impossible, did Vespasian's stubbornness relent. Now he spat, and rubbed the paralyzed limbs, and the blind saw, and the paralytic arose and walked.

§6. **Church Sleep.**—When, subsequently, the ancient religions died out, and had left the world as an heritage to Christianity, temple sleep had by no means died out also. On the contrary, after the lapse of three centuries, it again came into favor with the Christian priests. And the use of it now was scarcely less in favor than it had been a thousand years previous in the world of the ancient Greeks. Let us mention a few examples. The first four stories are taken from the works of Gregory of Tours.

Mummolus, who came to the court of Justinian (527 to 565) as the ambassador of King Theudebert, suffered greatly from calculi of the urinary bladder, and during this journey he became subject to an attack of renal colic. Things went badly with poor Mummolus, and he was in a great hurry to make his will. Whereupon he was advised to pass one night sleeping in St. Andrew's Church, at Pateras, for St.Andrew had performed many miraculous cures in this place. No sooner said than done. Mummolus, greatly tormented by pain and fever, and despairing of life, had himself placed upon the stone flags of the sanctuary, and waited there for the things that were to happen. Suddenly, toward midnight, the patient awoke with a violent desire to urinate, and discharged in a natural manner a calculus which, as St.Gregory assures us, was so enormous that it fell with a loud clatter into the vessel. From that hour Mummolus was hale and hearty, and joyfully started on his journey homeward.

In Brioude, the capital of the present department Haute-Loire, there was a woman named Fedamia, who had been paralyzed for years. In addition to this, she was penniless, and her relatives, therefore, brought her to the Church of St. Julian, who enjoyed a great reputation in Brioude, in order that, even if she did not become cured, she might at least make some money by begging at the church door. For eighteen years she had lived thus when, one Sunday night, while she slept in the colonnade adjoining the church, a man appeared who took her by the hand and led her toward the grave of St. Julian. On arriving there she uttered a fervent prayer, and in a moment felt as if a load of actual chains fell from her limbs. All this, it is true, happened in a dream, but when the patient awoke she was hale and hearty, and was able, to the amazement of the assembled multitude, to walk, with loud prayers, to the grave of the saint.

A certain man, deaf, dumb, and blind, known by the name of Amagildus, also tried the sleep in the Church of St. Julian, at Brioude. But it appears that this saint was not always quite accessible to the wishes of the sick. It is true, Amagildus was not obliged, like Fedamia of the previous narrative, to pass eighteen years in the basilica, but, nevertheless, he had to sleep for a full year in the colonnade of the church before the curative power of the holy martyr delivered him from his ailment.

Veranus, the slave of one of the clergy under Gregory, was so violently attacked by gout that he was absolutely unable to move for an entire year. Thereupon his master pledged himself to advance the afflicted slave to the priesthood if St. Martin would be willing to cure him. To accomplish this cure the slave was carried to the church, and there placed at the feet of the saint. The poor wretch had to remain there for five long days, and it seemed as tho St. Martin had forgotten all about him. Finally, on the sixth day, the patient was visited by a man who seized his foot and drew it out straight. The slave rose to his feet in terror, and perceived that he was cured. For many years he served St. Martin as a priest.

But the most wonderful cure was that of the German emperor Henry II., called "The Saint" (1002 to 1024). This emperor, who was of Bavarian stock, suffered greatly from the stone, and had retired to the Italian cloister Monte Cassino, inasmuch as this cloister during that period justly enjoyed an extraordinary medical reputation. But whether the monks of Monte Cassino, altho well versed in medical art, did not have sufficient confidence in their ability to treat an emperor, or whether they were induced by some other reason, is not known; however, instead of submitting the imperial patient to the operations of terrestrial medicine, they surrendered him to the providence of heaven, and more particularly to the sympathy of St. Benedict. This saint fully justified the confidence that was placed in him, for, during an acute period in the patient's sufferings, he appeared in his own holy person, and with his own holy hands he performed the necessary operation, and, after having pressed the stone that he had removed from the bladder into the hand of the sleeping emperor, he retired heavenward. But he took care from his heavenly residence to attend to the prompt healing of the operation wound, and this was surely very good of St.Benedict. In fact, his entire behavior during this case was extremely proper and laudable; for is it not much more fitting that the imperial bladder should be delivered from its disagreeable visitor, the stone, at the hands of a saint than by those of mortal beings, even if those mortal beings were the pious and medically skilled monks of Monte Cassino?[3]

---

[3] Compare Leibnitz, Script. Brunsvic, Vol. I., page 525. Sprengel, Vol. II., page 91.

The form in which we encounter the Christian temple sleep in the above stories is as like as two peas to that practised in the Hellenic temples. They are distinguished merely by the fact that the Greek gods generally hastened to the assistance of the patients after the latter had spent one night in the temple, whereas the Christian saints often allowed years to pass before the patient, who was crying for aid, secured relief.

Christianity has, however, created one variation of the temple sleep, and this is the sleep which is taken, altho outside of the church, at any place whatever, but with invocation of the saints. This sleep was said to be exactly as efficacious as that taken in the church itself, provided the patient had fervently prayed before falling asleep, and had particularly remembered the saint whose assistance he required. The two following narratives, which are also taken from the works of Gregory of Tours, may serve as significant examples of this variety of temple sleep.

Alpinus, Count of Tours, was so tormented for years by a pain in his foot that life had no further joys for him, so that, sleepless and without appetite, he took to his bed. Again and again had he, in secret prayer, appealed to St. Martin for relief. So one day the Count suddenly falls into a deep sleep, during which St. Martin appears to him, making the sign of the cross over the diseased foot. Thereupon the pain suddenly left him, and Alpinus was able to leave his couch, fully cured. In this case the saint showed himself extremely considerate toward the sick count, in that he was attired in a smart uniform when paying his visit. It was his intention, obviously, in choosing this costume to gratify the martial tastes of the nobleman; for St. Martin, when visiting patients, by no means always affected this warlike array, as will be seen from the following story.

A certain woman was so severely afflicted with campsis of the fingers that she completely lost the use of her hands. Even a visit to the church which was consecrated to St. Martin in Tours had brought her no relief. The patient was obliged to leave the sanctuary with her fingers still diseased. But it seems that this patient was actually of a very contented disposition; for when, upon her return, away from Tours, she lay down to her first night's rest, she thanked God that at least her life was spared, and that she had been permitted to see the grave of St. Martin. Affected by so much modesty, St. Martin appeared to her in her sleep, and, like to St. Benedict in the case of the emperor Henry, with his own holy hands he performed somewhat of an operation upon the patient, in that he stretched her bent fingers in such a manner that the tense tendons were evidently torn; for Gregory tells us that, under the treatment described, blood flowed from the straightened fingers of the woman. But St. Martin had entirely discarded his martial attire upon this visit. Evidently such a garb did not seem to him appropriate when visiting a female patient; he therefore appeared before the patient in a purple cloak with a cross in his hand.

However, the medical activity of the saints was by no means restricted to cases of church slumber, but was manifested in the most various forms.

§ 7. **Medical Saints.**—Some saints had a decided predilection for medical specialties, and for that reason paid a particular attention to certain varieties of disease. Thus, St. Anna espoused ophthalmology;St. Jude cured coughs; St. Valentine, epilepsy; St. Catherine of Siena, the plague. Not even our domestic animals were forgotten by the saints. Thus, St. Roch of Montpellier distinguished himself especially by his skill as a veterinarian.

Various were the ways of obtaining the medical aid of this or that saint. The most simple was probably that the patient attended mass in the church of his town, and, at the same time, made an offering to the saints. More difficult was it to undertake a pilgrimage to one or the other of the saints who enjoyed a medical reputation; this was generally done on the birthday of the celestial physician. It seems that the saint was especially inclined on this day to practise medicine; at least, the chroniclers report that great numbers of the most difficult cases were successfully treated on such days.

A very efficacious method of securing medical treatment from saints was considered to be the placing of the patient in the church during the day in the space between the altar and the grave of the saint. The bed of the mortally sick, fever-racked patient was placed there, and for days was compelled to remain here wrestling with death. This was done, for instance, with the dying Countess Eborin. In case severe epidemics were prevalent, it is likely that the churches very often resembled actual hospitals. Then dozens of beds with their patients were set up in the churches, and many a one who was in good health when he entered the church to say his prayers probably returned home with the germ of a pestilence acquired in the sanctuary.

But the saints, as we have seen, were by no means always so anxious or in such a hurry to manifest their medical skill. They often made the patient wait for years for their aid. The church, therefore, made practical arrangements to meet every requirement. Larger buildings were erected close to the church intended for the reception of patients. Here those who were hoping to find help could obtain shelter and food, and were, therefore, able to rest quietly, and to await the moment when heavenly aid might appear. This arrangement proved to be extremely practical, especially because a good many individuals felt themselves cured only so long as they remained in the proximity of the saint, but became reafflicted as before when they returned to their homes.

But as the slumber and the protracted sojourn in the ecclesiastical hostelries was, nevertheless, rather uncomfortable, especially in consideration of the difficulties and dangers which were involved in traveling during the middle ages, it was absolutely necessary to invent a means of administering the medical aid of the saints in such a way as was always accessible to the patient. This was managed by the use of relics.

§8. **Cult of Relics.**—It was believed that God had endowed the bodies of martyrs who died for the Christian faith, or of saints distinguished by extraordinary piety, with a miraculous power of

60

extraordinary efficacy, and not only the mortal relics of the martyrs and saints were wonder-working, but actually all objects which had come in contact with the persons of saints during their life as well as after their death. All such objects were possessed of curative power. Let us listen to what Gregory of Tours says under this head: "The miracles which our Lord God deigned to bring about through St. Martin, his servant, once a pilgrim in the flesh, he causes to be repeated daily, to strengthen the confidence of the faithful; for now he endows his tomb with precisely the same wonder-working power as was exhibited by the saint himself while still among us. Who will now persist in doubting the former miracles when he observes their continuation in the present day, when he sees the lame walk, the blind receive their sight, devils cast out, and every variety of disease cured by the help of the saint?" ("Bernoulli," page 287).

The statement of such a luminary of the Church as Gregory of Tours has undoubtedly gained ecclesiastical credence for the medical efficacy not only of the tomb of St. Martin, but of all the relics relating to that saint. It remained only to distribute the superior medical power which was contained in the holy tombs and relics in such a form as would enable all patients, wherever they happened to be, to make use of them. This task, apparently most difficult, was settled very easily. It was discovered that everything which came in contact with a relic actually absorbed a sacred and miraculous power contained in the same, and what had been absorbed was by no means imponderable. Quite the contrary. Something of material substance, and, therefore, physically demonstrable, passed from the relic into the objects surrounding it. It was indeed a celestial fluid, but, nevertheless, of so terrestrial a nature that the priests were able to demonstrate its transference by means of a common pair of scales. Thus it was customary that the silk shreds which were deposited by the pilgrims upon the tomb of the apostle Peter were weighed before they were placed there and weighed again after their removal. This weighing always and without exception indicated a considerable increase in their weight. The pilgrim then could travel homeward and be thoroughly consoled, as the scale had demonstrated to him the amount of miraculous power contained in his silk rag. It was really astonishing, under some circumstances, what an enormous amount of curative fluid could flow from such a holy tomb into a single terrestrial object. This was what happened to a king of the Suavians. He had a sick son, for whose cure every remedy had proved unavailing. He at last sent an embassy to Tours to obtain a relic of St. Martin, but this relic was destined to be manufactured with the assistance of the embassy. The priests were quite willing to comply with the desire of their royal petitioner, and thus a piece of silk, duly weighed beforehand, was placed upon the tomb of St. Martin. After this silk had remained for one night upon the holy sepulchre, and the embassy had knelt beside praying fervently, the silk absorbed so much curative power that the register of the scale was raised to its highest possible notch.

Knowing, then, that any desired object could be saturated with the miraculous power contained in a relic, they used to apply this celestial power through medicaments, and to accomplish this a number of methods were in use. The most popular was to scrape the tombstones on the graves of the saints as thoroughly as possible. The powder thus obtained was then put into water or wine, and thus a medicine was acquired which possessed an astonishing curative power. It was efficacious even in the severest ailments of the body. Let us listen to what Gregory of Tours has reported concerning the medicinal virtues of such tombstone potions.

He says: "Oh, indescribable mixture, incomparable elixir, antidote beyond all praise! Celestial purgative (if I may be permitted to use the expression), which throws into the shade every medical prescription, which surpasses in fragrance every earthly aroma, and is more powerful than all essences; which purges the body like the juice of scammony, clears the lungs like hyssop, and the head like sneezewort; which not only cures the ailing limbs, but also, and this is much more valuable, washes off the stains from the conscience!"

According to this extensive power of the tombstone powder, it is by no means astonishing that Gregory of Tours, when traveling, always carried a box of this miraculous powder with him, so that he was able at once to heal the patients that surrounded him. I was not able to obtain from the literary sources at my disposal any data as to whether the direct licking off of the tombstones might not have been still more efficacious than the all-healing extract. Gregory does, however, report that he was cured of a tumor of the tongue and lips by merely licking the railing of the tomb of St. Martin and kissing the curtain of the temple.

Another very efficacious remedy was the charred wick of the wax candles which had burned in the church. This wick was pulverized, and in this manner a very powerful curative powder was obtained which, when taken, acted in a manner similar to that of the watery or vinous tombstone infusion.

The wax which dripped from candles that were placed near the holy sepulchre was also credited with many medicinal virtues, but it seems that it was employed more as an external than an internal remedy.

The water which had been used before Easter to clean the altar of the saints was also considered to be a famous remedy. If such water was employed in washing a patient he recovered at once, and this was the happy experience of Countess Eborin. This exhalted patient was suffering so severely that she believed her hour had come. She was then quickly removed to the church of St. Martin, and thoroughly washed with the water that had been used in washing the altar. And, behold! the disease disappeared, and let us hope that the overjoyed countess afterward enjoyed many years of life.

Oil from lamps hung in holy places was also a favorite remedy, but it appears that it was principally used for anointing. However, when mixed with holy water, it furnished a remedy which could be administered to diseased cattle with a prospect of positive cure.

Water which was obtained by boiling the covers in which the relics were wrapped also yielded a very efficacious medicine. Thus, for instance, Gregory of Tours caused a silk cover, in which a piece of the cross of Christ had been wrapped, to be thoroughly boiled, and he then administered this decoction to patients; the curtains which were used as ornaments over holy graves also displayed an extremely beneficent effect upon the sick. If an individual suffering from headache touched, for instance, the carpet which was placed over the resting-place of St. Julian, the pain ceased. But if a patient was afflicted with abdominal pains, all that was necessary to relieve him at once was to pull a thread from this, the above-named carpet, and to apply it to his rebellious digestive apparatus.

However, it was not necessary for the priests, under some circumstances, personally to take the trouble of manufacturing miraculous medicines from relics. There existed some holy graves which were so accommodating that they furnished, of their own accord, the holy material that was required for the treatment of the sick. Thus the chronicler records that the grave of the evangelist John exuded a sort of white manna, which, owing to its wonder-working curative power, was distributed all over the world. A similar product was yielded by the grave of the Apostle Andrew on the festival day of that saint. A precious oil scented like nectar also sprang from the resting-place of this man of God.

We see, therefore, that the sacred pharmacopœia teemed with remedies, and that they were quite extensively employed is shown sufficiently by the history of the saints and, above all, by the works of Gregory of Tours. The latter, in particular, offer an actually inexhaustible mine of information concerning the medical activity of Christian saints.

It does not, however, appear that this medical activity enjoyed the confidence of priests or of laymen to such an extent that the services of a professional physician were entirely discarded. It is true, Gregory of Tours expresses himself in reference to the terrestrial physicians in a manner which is by no means complimentary, for he says:

"What are they (the physicians) able to accomplish with their instruments? Their office is rather to cause pain than to alleviate it; if they open the eye and cut into it with pointed lancets, they surely cause the agony of death to come in sight before assisting in the recovery of vision, and if all precautionary measures are not thoroughly carried out the power of sight is lost forever. Our beloved saint, however, has only one instrument of steel, and that is his will, and only one salve, and that is his curative power."

But in spite of this want of confidence in physicians, Gregory of Tours did not hesitate eventually to interfere quite extensively with the practise of the saints by the employment of ordinary medicine.

At least, he frequently did so when he felt sick himself. Thus, one day, when he was afflicted with severe bellyache, he employed warm poultices and

66

baths, and only when the refractory abdomen gave him no rest, after a continuance of this treatment for six days, did Gregory apply to St. Martin. When, at another time, Gregory was affected with so severe an attack that his death was believed to be imminent, he caused himself at first to be treated according to all the rules of medical science, and not until improvement failed to appear, did he think of the aid of the saints. Then he spoke to his physician as follows: "Well, you have exhausted all remedies of your art, you have used up all your powers and juices, but the remedies of this world do not help him who is destined to die. Only one thing remains for me to do. I shall tell you the great remedy: take some stone powder from the grave of St. Martin and prepare it for me."

The healing of the sick by the power of the saints and through relics was in favor throughout the middle ages, and even in the sixteenth century it was so generally in vogue that a physician by the name of Wyer (1515 to 1588) considered it expedient to demonstrate the incredibility of such heavenly interference.

It is by no means my intention to hold solely dogmatic Christendom of the middle ages and the Christian priest responsible for the monstrous superstition into which, according to the above description, Christian religion had degenerated in the domain of medicine. This superstition resulted from the cooperation of quite incongruous factors; but we can by no means exempt the Christian priest entirely from blame, in that he assisted very materially in furthering it. For we must bear in mind that the Christian cloister of the middle ages was not only the last refuge of humanistic culture, but the science of medicine found an asylum of preeminent importance within its precincts. Medicine had taken refuge in the cloister from the storms and tribulations which followed the political collapse of antiquity and from the excitement of national migrations, and had here attained a high degree of perfection. In fact, we may contend, without exaggeration, that at certain periods of the middle ages the Christian monastery had the importance as a medical school which was later on claimed by the university; for the Christian monks not only nursed the sick and practised medicine, but also took an interest in its scientific development. They were well acquainted with the medical classics of ancient times, such as Hippocrates, Herophilus, Dioscorides, Galen, Paul of Ægina, and others, as well as with the ancient medical celebrities of second and third rank. Briefly, medical knowledge in its entirety was contained in the cloisters of the middle ages; the cloisters, indeed, furnished a considerably larger quota of the medical profession than the laity. In such a state of affairs it might have been expected that the monks and priests should have applied their extensive medical knowledge to combat the terrible abuses which had invaded medicine in connection with the names and the bones of the saints. But this they never did, neither during the middle ages or later on. Priesthood has never seriously attempted to promote medical enlightenment. On the contrary, plenty of writings exist in which the crassest superstition in medico-physical affairs was defended by the clergy, who quite frequently exhibit the same spirit while practising medicine. Medical relief obtained by entirely terrestrial remedies they speedily placed to the credit of the saints, as was done, for instance, by the monks of Monte Cassino, when (as we have seen above) they persuaded the emperor Henry II. that not the temporal hands of the friar physicians had performed an operation for stone upon him, but that St.Benedict in person had, with his own holy hands, extracted the stone from the imperial bladder.

By leading the laity, in numerous cases and against their better knowledge and conscience, to believe that the aid of the saints, and of the relics originating from them, was far superior to medical services, the Christian priests of the middle ages have on their part contributed quite a considerable share to the horrors of medical superstition. It is true, we must not overlook the fact that monks and priests of the middle ages were the product of their time, in the same manner as we of modern times are the product of our period. And as the middle ages formed an era of miracles, of demons, devils, and witches, numerous members of the clergy, as children of their time, surely had an essentially different opinion of the belief in miracles and demons from that which we have. The conception of miracles was entirely different during the middle ages from what it is in modern times; for the sincere and firm belief in the omnipotence of the one God, which with Christianity had taken possession of the world, had firmly fixed in the Christian mind of that period the idea that God was able at any moment to manifest his omnipotence by changing the course of terrestrial phenomena, and actually did manifest it. Thus to a Christian of the middle ages it did not appear miraculous that an alteration in the course of natural law should occur. It was considered quite conceivable that the same natural phenomena should spring from one cause to-day and from a different one to-morrow, according to the pleasure of God; it would have been just as inconceivable to the early Christians, and to their later coreligionists of the middle ages, that all natural processes are carried into effect according to eternally unalterable laws, beyond the interference of divinity, as it is incomprehensible to us to conceive that God would at any time change a law of nature in favor of one or the other mortal being. The conception of miracle during the first sixteen centuries of the Christian era was entirely different from that of the subsequent era. We must not, therefore, gauge the ideas of priests and laymen of those centuries who believed in medical miracles by the same standard as that by which we judge those who to-day still persist in admitting the existence of medico-physical wonder or miracle. It is highly probable that, under conditions as described above, many Christian monks and priests vacillated between the requirements of faith and the results of their own medical knowledge. The medieval scholar's feeling drew him to one side, his intelligence to the other, and thus he became destitute of a firm hold—the intellectual sport of his period and of his environment. That prominent lights of the Church could become subject to such vacillations we learn from Gregory of Tours, who attempted to cure bodily ailments at one time with the medicaments of professional medicine, at other times with the saving means of the celestial drug-store; who at one time deprecated the art of temporal physicians in favor of medically skilled saints, at other times fled to human medicine for refuge.

Finally the position of the medically learned monk and priest with reference to the general public, during the middle ages, was by no means an easy or an agreeable one. The people clung with invincible tenacity to the belief in demons and miracles. Ancient as well as Christian philosophy was firmly pledged to a belief in demons, whose existence was supported by the sacred testimony of the Gospel. It is not astonishing, therefore, that the people should cling to their belief in various forms of supernatural interference with the functions of organic beings, and thus it may frequently have happened that a medically enlightened priest, fearing the opposition of a people eager after celestial medicine, sacrificed his scientific convictions to the caprices of a mistaken faith. Unfortunately, only a few had in them the making of a scientific martyr, and the history of Christianity teaches us that it is much easier to be a martyr of faith than a martyr of science.

But what has been stated thus far will by no means acquit the Christian priest of blame which he incurred by favoring medical superstition; such acquittal would be radically futile. But we mean to show that the conduct of the servants of our faith, altho not pardonable, is quite explicable. The historian, in order to present to his readers the relation which had gradually formed between Christianity and medical superstition, must show himself prosecutor and defendant at the same time.

Equally with dogma and priesthood, theistic belief also has been a powerful instrument in the furthering of medical superstition, and this point we shall next consider.

§9. **Theistic Thought as the Fosterer of Medical Superstition.**—Altho the theist, by accepting a physico-mechanical interpretation of natural phenomena, abandoned his main position, yet the theistic belief by no means became obsolete—i.e., the belief that God, unrestricted by natural laws, personally directed terrestrial manifestations still held its ground. This belief remained dominant in many minds, in spite of all that philosophers and naturalists said in regard to the forms and life of organic structures. The vitality which this belief has shown during the development of our race is actually astonishing. In spite of the wide acceptance of the physico-mechanical theory of life, the belief that God, without regard to natural laws, unceasingly interfered with the course of natural events, and, consequently, also with the conditions of the human body, has not only remained active, but has even succeeded in recovering an extensive part of its lost ground. We shall soon see that this is a repetition of what has occurred during all periods of human development. Even to-day, when the mechanical theory of life has won its greatest triumphs, and more than twenty centuries have passed since the great Hippocrates preached a theory of medicine, purified from all theistic and theurgic accretions, individuals are still met with who presuppose the therapeutic activity of God in all cases of disease as a self-evident fact. Such a condition of opinion, history teaches us, always prevails at periods, during which a craving for religious excitement becomes excessively acute. It is either a new form of religion which so preoccupies the public mind and the intelligence that all phenomena are conceived of as in closest relationship with God, or else some individual appears who, carried away by religious enthusiasm, teaches that the existence of nature independent of God is not admissible, and succeeds in enlisting numerous followers under his banner. Under similar conditions theistic belief had occasionally succeeded in regaining its supremacy in the domain of medicine. In taking up the consideration of some such instances we can only treat them briefly, as an exhaustive handling of this most interesting material would carry us too far away from our present subject.

The belief that God was the best physician, not only of the soul but of the body also, was deepened by the dissemination of Christianity. The sincerity of faith among the Christians of the first century was so intense that a great number of them believed that their bodily welfare could not be watched over more carefully than when it was commended exclusively to the care of God in all cases of sickness. Accordingly, they entirely neglected medical aid and treated all diseases only by prayers, by anointing, and by laying on of hands. This mode of treatment corresponds to what is contained in the epistle of James v : 14-16—

"Is any sick among you? let him call for the elders of the church; and let them pray over him, anointing him with oil in the name of the Lord:

"And the prayer of faith shall save the sick, and the Lord shall raise him up; and if he have committed sins, they shall be forgiven him.

"Confess your faults one to another, and pray one for another, that ye may be healed. The effectual fervent prayer of a righteous man availeth much."

The extent of this treatment by prayer is shown by the fact that even prominent fathers of the Church—for instance, St. Benedict (died 543)—were addicted to it.

Moreover, an attempt was made to increase the therapeutic value of prayer by various accessories and aids. Thus the Gospel was placed upon the affected part of the body, or clothing of a particularly pious man was spread over the patient. It appears that the sudarium and the coat of the apostle Paul were held to possess such healing power, and were, therefore, frequently employed as instruments of healing. Thus we read in the Act of the Apostles xix : 12—"So that from his body were brought unto the sick handkerchiefs or aprons, and the diseases departed from them, and the evil spirits went out of them."

In fact, medical superstition went so far that it divined a potent curative virtue even in the shadow of the apostle Peter. Thus, Acts v : 15—"Insomuch that they brought forth the sick into the streets, and laid them on beds and couches, that at least the shadow of Peter passing by might overshadow some of them."

Probably we shall not be wrong in regarding this procedure as the origin of that relic cult which was destined to attain such astonishing dimensions in medical practise.

The mode of treatment by means of prayer was, perhaps, intimately connected with the idea that bodily ailments were divinely ordained to make the wrath of God distinctly perceptible by man. This conception of pathological processes was a very ancient one. We meet with it among the Egyptians, and we read in the book of Exodus that God visited upon Pharaoh and his people various bodily afflictions, such as pestilence, black smallpox, death, as in the case of the first-born. Afterward Christianity adopted this view of sickness as providential, and the belief assumed very peculiar forms and dimensions in the middle ages. In those times any disease occurring epidemically was actually considered to be an act of retribution on the part of the divine being, a scourge with which God punished sinful Christians. Thus, for instance, syphilis, which originated in Naples in 1495, during the struggle between the reigning house of Aragon and the French, was instantly declared to be the chastisement of God. The emperor Maximilian declares, in an edict issued August 7, 1495, at Worms: *"Quod novus ille et gravissimus hominum morbus nostris diebus exortus, quem vulgo malum Francicum vocant, post hominum memoriam inauditus sæpe grassetur, quæ nos justissimæ Dei iræ merita debent admonere*" (Gregorovius VII., 386, foot-note 1).

But it is very astonishing to observe the causes which aroused the wrath of God so mightily that countless numbers of men were swept away. Thus, for instance, the pious Bishop of Zeeland, Peter Paladius, assures us that miliary fever, that terrible disease which devastated Europe five times from 1486 to 1551, was sent by God, who was angry at the excessive passion for finery which prevailed at that time. Medical science, as founded on theism, assumed menacing forms, where, in the middle ages, it associated itself with magic, but as we shall more exhaustively enlarge upon this point in Chapter IV. we need merely refer here to that part of our work.

It is indeed surprising that the above-mentioned manifestations all occurred in periods in which medicine had already acknowledged the physico-mechanical interpretation of all organic processes; but the strangeness of this fact is enhanced by the consideration that, even in recent times, and even at the present moment, there have been, and are, individuals who not only preach the doctrine that medicine is bound to be subordinate to Christian faith, but also find adherents to their dogmas, and find them in surprising numbers. Recently we have learned from two exceedingly instructive examples to what extremes the sentiment of fanatical religion may lead men so soon as they shake off the steadying influence of physico-mechanical ideas in their theory of life. Then Theocracy strives for an exclusive ascendancy in the domain of medicine, as is distinctly shown by the position taken by Mrs. Eddy, with her "Christian Science," and Rev. John Alexander Dowie, with his "Christian Catholic Church of Zion."

If we first of all examine the system of Mrs. Eddy, we find it an absurd farrago of undigested philosophical odds and ends, illogical medical aphorisms, and shallow investigation, which reaches its pitch of folly in the belief that disease has no real foundation in the material tissues of the body, but should be explained as arising exclusively from certain conditions of the mind. In accordance with this conception, which has been borrowed from a natural philosophy long since relegated to oblivion, the services both of physician and physic are to be rejected, and the treatment of the sick is to be carried on in such a manner that the patient, under supervision of an individual expert in such affairs, is merely to fix his mind on the spiritual, or divine, principle inherent in himself.

We are by no means astonished that a person to whom the laws of thought are entirely unfamiliar, and who is not very much burdened with knowledge of any other kind, should advance such confused and preposterous theories as those of Mrs. Eddy. History teaches us that human beings have arisen at all periods, in all ranks of life, and in cold blood have given currency to the wildest of theories. But the most interesting point is that at this day when, as we might believe, the advances in physical science have enlightened to some extent even the most unintellectual, Mrs. Eddy is able to find adherents, especially among the best classes of society, and to find them in such numbers that the authorities have been compelled to interfere in repressing the practises of this medical superstition. I purposely say interesting, and not "astonishing" or "wonderful," because the historian, whatever domain he undertakes to investigate, will always discover that stupidity has at all times been a power superior to all the influences of culture and learning. Mrs. Eddy, with her Christian Science, proves to us that even in this era of scientific enlightenment, this truth remains incontrovertible.

Rev. John Alexander Dowie, with his Christian Catholic Church of Zion, must be judged from an entirely different view-point than Mrs. Eddy. It is true, this latter-day saint arrives at exactly the same end as Mrs. Eddy—namely, at the absolute rejection of professional treatment, medical as well as surgical. But he arrives at this theory, which so closely concerns both his own health and that of his adherents, by an entirely different way from that taken by the Eddy woman. An unquestioning belief, which in its naïveté is almost touching, leads him to hold that all utterances of the Old as well as of the New Testament are direct revelations of God. The further consequence of this constancy of faith is the desire to believe and to follow everything that is contained in the Bible, to the widest extent and with the closest adherence to the wording of the book. And as the book of Exodus, xv : 26, states, "I am the Lord that healeth thee," and in the Epistle to James, v : 14-16, prayer is recommended as the best remedy in diseases, Dowie concludes that prayer must be resorted to as the sole means of treating and curing all forms of disease. Prayer is declared by him to be much more efficacious, in surgical cases, than the skill of the most experienced operator.

Dowie, therefore, occupies exactly the same standpoint as the Christians of the first centuries after Christ, who also believed that prayer would render the best assistance in all ailments of the body. Twenty centuries, therefore, with all their immense advance in the training of thought and in the recognition of nature, have not been able to rid humanity of the conception that the omnipotence of God, among many other manifestations, is to busy itself in the daily regulation of the human body with all its numerous functions. Wherever this conception obtains a firm foothold superstition, with its acts of miraculous healing, never fails to follow. Accordingly, all historic periods of our cultural development, in which the theocratic belief has been on the ascendant, are characterized by an excessive development of medical superstition.

IV

THE INFLUENCE OF PHILOSOPHY UPON THE FORM AND ORIGIN OF MEDICAL SUPERSTITION

THE idea that philosophy has exerted any material influence upon superstition in medicine may appear strange to many. For how can it be possible that the science which teaches the laws of thought, which regulates our entire mental activity and guides it in the right direction, which points out to us the intricate path of medical theory and diagnosis—how is it possible that just this science should either take or have taken part in misleading or obscuring our medical perception? We do not by any means intend to impute any such effect to philosophy. Quite the contrary! We are thoroughly aware of the great influence which philosophy is entitled to claim in all sciences without exception, and for this reason we believe that modern representatives of medical science would be much better off if they were a little less at variance with philosophy than they actually are.

In the wide realm of philosophy there are only certain points where we can detect a tendency to promote the development of medical superstition. This tendency appears in all endeavors which are made to explain natural phenomena solely in a speculative manner, or to build a theory of life upon a base of pure assumptions. Whenever such attempts were made manifest, and impressed philosophy into their service under the name of natural philosophy, it resulted in the wide predominance of medical superstition.

It is well known that all prae-Socratic philosophy aimed at the discovery of a single principle as underlying and explaining all the phenomena of nature. But in spite of this very apparent tendency, it can scarcely be accused of promoting medical superstition; for prae-Socratic philosophy busied itself in speculations concerning terrestrial phenomena. Earth and air, fire and water, cold and heat, coming into being and passing away, are the things in which it endeavored to find the elemental basis of nature with its multiform phenomena. But upon the study of medicine these endeavors exercised, for the time being, a liberalizing influence. They emancipated it from the repressive grasp of theism, and opened up the way for an exclusively natural explanation of all processes of the body, in health as well as in sickness. Unfortunately the apparatus, or organon, which philosophy furnished to science in its terrestrial phenomena was a very questionable one, investigation of the conclusion from analogy and the deductive method being of extremely little value, either in medical diagnosis or the pursuit of natural science. For this reason medicine was bound to be encumbered with countless badly founded hypotheses. But other monstrous guesses at truth could not fail to become current. Let us consider, for instance, the absurd theory which Heraclitus of Ephesus (500 B.C.) has propounded as to the relations between wine and the human soul. As the soul, according to this philosopher, naturally was a fiery vapor, and the drier and the more fiery it remained the better, the excessive use of alcohol would not be advisable, in that the abundant infusion of fluids causes the soul to become wet, which would be harmful to its fiery nature, as fire and moisture are always incompatible. Who will venture to deny that it was from his opinion regarding the use of wine that Heraclitus acquired his sobriquet of "Whining Philosopher"?

But curious as were all the hypotheses with which Hellenic natural philosophy foisted upon medicine, they should by no means be confounded with superstition, for even a baseless hypothesis is far removed from superstition. Otherwise, medicine and superstition would be almost identical conceptions, for baseless hypotheses have at no time been wanting in our science. Superstition, so far as its sources are found in philosophy, did not enter medical science until philosophy sought for an explanation of the various processes of life not only in material but also in immaterial forces. And as Indian as well as Persian philosophy, in the earliest period of its existence known to us, had already found in demons the immaterial elements which to a great extent control the processes of life in man, it will be seen that the relations between philosophy and medical superstition are quite old. The Hellenic poets and philosophers, Homer, Hesiod, Empedocles, Democritus, and Plato, elaborated this immemorial doctrine of demons and introduced it into Greece. But the recognition of immaterial, supernatural curative factors did not attain any considerable and determining influence in ancient medicine until the year 150 B.C., when, under the eager advocacy of Alexandrian Jews, Oriental and Occidental doctrines became amalgamated to a coherent system of theosophic and medical mysticism. Medicine suffered greatly for centuries from this mysticism, which prevailed late in the middle ages and even up to more recent times. The center of all the various forms under which speculations in the philosophical and theosophical domain made their appearance was Alexandria, the great central point of culture in which the civilization of the Orient and the Occident were united in the evolution of a new theory of life. But that the birthplace of developments so momentous for the future of medicine should be Alexandria almost suggests the thought that the writers of history were indulging in a satire upon medical science; for it is well known that Alexandria was the very place where medical enlightenment and the progress of ancient medicine won their greatest triumphs under the renowned anatomists, Herophilus and Erasistratus.

Such speculations in theosophical and medical domains at first were most eagerly entered upon by the Jewish sects of the Essenians, or Essenes, and Therapeutæ. According to the description which Josephus (Book 2, Chapter II., page 13) has left us of these two sects, they were theosophical communists. We, as physicians, however, are principally interested in the position they took with regard to our profession, and that was one of indifference. They believed that they should not obtain their knowledge of the body, either in health or in disease, by observation, on which physicians relied. They believed they could actually learn the art of healing from a study of their old Sacred Scriptures. For that reason they especially applied themselves to make a diligent examination of these Holy Scriptures. They believed that they were able, by various allegorical interpretations of different letters and words, as well as by subtle explanations of this or that sentence, to acquire the knowledge necessary for the treatment of their patients. Those, however, who had become imbued with this wisdom of dotage in an especial degree, claimed the possession of numerous miraculous powers—for instance, that of prediction. But as they also believed in the existence of beings who, while they were lower than God, at the same time were higher than man, they had, ready at hand, the rarest resources to draw upon for the practise of their juggling feats of miraculous medicine. The belief in these mystical doctrines took the most extravagant forms. Thus, for instance, it was believed that a man by the evacuation of feces offered an insult to divinity (τὰς αὐγὰς ὑβρίζειν τοῦ θεοῦ, says Josephus, lib. 2, Chapter VIII., No. 9, § 15). For that reason nobody might dare, on the Sabbath, to comply with such demands of nature. But whether the call of nature always yielded tothese rather far-reaching requirements of the law, or how the believer helped himself when the extremely disagreeable dissension between nature and faith caused too much uneasiness, is not reported either by Josephus or by Porphyrius. Besides, the Essenians had their troubles even on week-days in attending to final phases of the digestive process, in that it was incumbent upon them to conceal the termination of the act of digestion from the view of the Supreme Being by covering themselves with a cloak.

Subsequently, during the first century of the Christian era, appeared Neo-Pythagorism, an attempt to combine monotheism with the ancient fantastic cult of subordinate gods and demons. Then followed a period of momentous importance for medicine; for the attempt to displace the physico-mechanical conception of corporeal phenomena by various ideas of theosophic caprice, and to bring therapeutics once more under the domination of the metaphysic methods, prevalent in the days when the theistic theory of life held undisputed sway in medicine and natural sciences, became more and more apparent. The Neo-Pythagoreans acted upon the principle that the practise of medicine was absolutely indispensable to the true philosopher, and that every one, therefore, provided he had attained the required fitness by his intercourse with demons, was able to act as a physician. It is quite obvious that such ideas were bound to pave the way for the most abominable abuse and superstitions, and, naturally, what the Neo-Pythagoreans offered as the art of healing to the patients was nothing but a mixture of mysterious customs, conjurations, and witchcraft. On the other hand, the followers of this school of philosophy did much to promote the bodily welfare of their fellow men, in that they urged them to lead a pure and temperate life, while they themselves appear to have adhered strictly to this régime.

The chief representative of Neo-Pythagorism was Apollonius, of Tyana, in Cappodocia, probably one of the most fantastic personages of all Greek and Roman antiquity. Venerated as a god by some of his contemporaries, such as Damis and Philostratus, his biographers, on account of his wisdom and of his extraordinary works, he is considered by others, on the other hand, as a magician engaged, like a common charlatan, in conjuring tricks. The opinions which posterity, down to modern times, has passed on Apollonius are of a similar nature. There are some who consider the Tyanian to be a crafty magician, whereas others declare that he is an important personality in the history of religion. Among these latter is Baur, who attempts to explain the life and the deeds of the wonder-working Neo-Pythagorean by citing as a parallel the impression created by Christianity upon some enlightened minds.

Personally, I consider this high estimate of a trickster to be perfectly absurd. Apollonius, as we meet him in the celebrated description of Philostratus, is a purely poetical idealization, prompted by a desire to delay the downfall of ancient religion, pointing to the reform which has been instituted in its moral tendencies (Gregorovius, page 413).

Apollonius flourished in the first Christian century, during the reigns of Nero and of the succeeding emperors up to Nerva, who appears to have been in very close relations with him. The accounts of Philostratus regarding the adventures of our hero, based as they are upon the early authorities accessible to him, absolutely create the impression that heathen antiquity meant in Apollonius to set a counterpart of Christ. According to ancient reports, a supernatural apparition visited his mother, apprizing her that she would bear a god, and after his death Apollonius appeared to his disciples to announce to them the immortality of the soul. The time between the birth and death of the Tyanian was spent by him in restless wanderings over the then known world. Wherever he went he conversed on the deepest subjects with priests and cultured laymen, and upon request he also performed miracles of various kinds. Naturally, we are only interested in the medical performances of the wandering philosopher, and of these he is credited with a considerable number. He cured the lame simply by stroking the affected limbs; with equal facility he gave sight to the blind—in fact, he even attended to obstetrical cases without fear and trepidation. For instance, when the husband of a woman who had borne seven children, but always with the greatest difficulty, came to Apollonius, sadly telling him that his wife was again in labor and nobody was able to help her, the man of miracles told him to be of good cheer. Without even examining the woman for a possible narrow pelvis, or for some other obstacle to birth, he simply advised the husband to procure, as soon as possible, a living hare, and, with this hare in his arms, to walk round and round the woman in labor, and then allow the hare to run away. This one sample of his medical activity is sufficient to characterize Apollonius as a charlatan of the most contemptible class. When we learn, further, that he raised the dead without any difficulty, nobody will probably accuse us of an unjust opinion if we pronounce this philosopher, who was revered as a god by the heathen, a magician of the worst kind.

In order duly to enhance his authority Apollonius arrogated to himself certain mysterious powers. Thus, he pretended that he was able to speak all languages without having ever learned them; in fact, this philological talent even extended to the languages of the animals, which he undertook to master. We are scarcely surprised to learn, when we consider the powers bestowed upon him, that he knew the future, and was thoroughly aware of what happened at the same time at the most distant parts of the world. He also endeavored to bear witness to his vocation as a man of God by his manner of living and of dressing. Thus he was always attired in white linen garments, and walked about with long, flowing hair, followed by his disciples. He never ate meat, never partook of wine, and disdained love. It would seem, however, that in the last particular he was not quite consistent— at least, various erotic adventures are related of him.

The manner in which Apollonius cast out a demon in India is extremely amusing. A woman came, lamenting and crying, to the medical miracle worker, and asked him to deliver her sixteen-year-old son from an evil spirit. Apollonius at once gave her a letter directed to the evil spirit which contained, as Philostratus emphasizes particularly, the most terrible threats against the good-for-nothing tormentor. But the biographer does not tell us whether the reading of this letter caused the demon to desist from his improper behavior.

But as even in a man of miracles the hour-glass of life finally is emptied, so also a time came when Apollonius realized that he must pay his last debt to nature. But the Tyanian knew how to surround even the act of dying with a halo of the extraordinary. As a matter or fact, he did not die; but one day—if it is permissible to employ a trivial expression in speaking of a demi-god—he evaporated without anybody knowing what had become of him. This evaporation occurred in the following manner. There was in Crete a temple of Dictynna so securely guarded by vicious dogs that no one dared to approach. This temple was entered by Apollonius, whom the furious dogs left unmolested; but, after the doors of the sanctuary had closed behind the Pythagorean, suddenly there resounded female voices singing from the depth of the temple: "Leave the earth! Go heavenward!" With these sounds and words Apollonius disappeared forever. Thus his last medical act was a sleight-of-hand performance, in that he even snapped his fingers at death.

The grateful heathen world of antiquity rendered divine honors to Apollonius. In his birth-place, Tyana, a temple was erected in his honor at imperial expense, and the priests everywhere erected statues to a philosopher who had left this world without dying; in fact, even the Emperor Alexander Severus set up an image of Apollonius in his *lararium*, or domestic chapel. And thus to medical superstition was accorded a triumph which no legitimate practitioner of any age has ever enjoyed.

These theosophic vagaries reached their climax in Neo-Platonism, which was founded toward the end of the second century of the Christian era by the Alexandrian porter, Ammonius (175 to 242), and was further elaborated by Plotinus (204 to 269). This religious, philosophical system is of very particular interest in the history of medicine in that, in the first place, it stands in direct opposition to the physico-mechanical conception of disease, and, explaining sickness from a theistic standpoint as a logical consequence, rejects the treatment of disease by professional physicians.

Now this theistic conception of disease was based primarily upon the assumption that the universe is filled with countless demons, spirits which, altho essentially superior to man, are inferior to God. Such a demon was supposed to be the "spiritus rector" of all terrestrial occurrences, especially all evil events were attributed to him. ὅτι αὐτοὶ αἴτιοι γιγνόμενοι τῶν Περὶ τὴν γῆν καθημάτων, οἷον λοιμῶν, ἀΦοριῶν, σεισμῶν, αὐχμῶν Καὶ τῶν ὁμοίων (Porphyrius de Abst., lib. 2, 40). As the demons played havoc with the condition of the human body, protection against them could not be expected from a professional physician, but only from some one well versed in all their tricks and devices, and, therefore, alone able to punish them thoroughly for their mischievous behavior. This taming of the demon could be accomplished in various ways. Porphyrius enumerates three methods of gaining an influence over the host of demons.

The first and principal method (theosophy) attempted to attain the most intimate union with God. Prayer, abstraction of all thought from things earthly, and absorption in God were supposed to be the means of participation in certain divine powers. An individual thus favored was enabled in a trice to restore health to incurable patients, such as the blind, the deaf, and the lame, and even the power of raising the dead was conferred upon him. However, the acquisition of such extraordinary powers demanded certain qualifications of a rather exacting and terrestrial character. It was incumbent upon such an applicant for these special gifts to abstain from the use of meat, and, above all, from the society of women. How many were deterred by these fastidious requirements from choosing the career of a famous man of miracles we do not know. Nothing is reported on this subject by the pillars of Neo-Platonism (as, Plotinus, Porphyrius, Damascius, Jamblichus), nor do they state whether they themselves absolutely abstained from meat and from the society of women.

Theurgy was the second method of counteracting the evil influence of demons. In this way good demons were urged by prayer and offerings to ward off disease or other misfortune.

By the third method (goety) attempts were made to dispel the evil demons by conjurations and various kinds of mystical mummery. These mysterious accessories consisted mostly in muttering any number of words as meaningless as possible. The more meaningless and the more unintelligible were these words the more efficacious—according to the assurance of Jamblichus—they would prove, especially when they were taken from Oriental languages. For, as Jamblichus says, the Oriental languages are the most ancient—therefore, the most agreeable to the gods. In such a manner words utterly nonsensical were drawled out at the bedside, and, for greater security, written on tablets to be hung round the neck of the patient. The magic word "abracadabra" enjoyed especial respect. To render its power certain it was written as many times as it has letters, omitting the last letter each time until only one remained, and placing the words in such a succession as to form an equilateral triangle. A tablet thus inscribed was worn around the neck of the sufferer as an amulet. It may be that this wonder-working word has arisen from the word "abraxas," with which the gnostic Basilides meant to designate the aggregate of the three hundred and sixty-five forms of revelation of divinity which he assumed to exist. Numerous other explanations are in vogue, however, with regard to this medical, magic term (compare Häser, Vol. I., page 433). Very ancient magic words which had originated in the earliest periods of Hellenism were revived. Thus, to banish disease, certain words were employed which were said to be derived from the temple of Artemis in Ephesus, and which read: ασχι, Κατάσχι, λίε, τετράε, δαμναμενεύς, αἴσσον. The meaning of these words, according to the explanation of the Pythagorean, Androcydes, was: darkness, light, earth, air, sun, truth. Besides, the attempt was made to obtain directly from the demons such magic words as were endowed with curative power. For such purposes small children were employed, in whom it was supposed that the demons preferred to be present, and expressed themselves through their mouths. Such children, therefore, played a similar part as does a medium with modern spiritualists. The senseless stuff babbled by such a child was considered the immediate manifestation of a demon, and was accordingly utilized to banish the demons which brought on disease. Moreover, the nonsensical practise which was carried on by the Neo-Platonists by letter and word was to a certain extent accepted by professional physicians. It had become a very common custom with physicians to apply various kinds of bombastic names to all their various plasters and ointments, powders, and pills. It is necessary only to cast a glance upon the ancient pharmacopœia to find the most curious names. Galen mentions disapprovingly the fact that Egyptian and Babylonian expressions were preferred in the nomenclature of medicine (De Simpl. Medicamentorum Facult. Lib. Sic. Preface).

Such were the methods with which the Neo-Platonists did not hesitate to treat the sick; and not only minor practitioners, but even the leaders of the entire movement, preferred banishing disease by means of various kinds of magic formulæ to all other specially medical methods of treatment. Thus, for instance, Eunapius of Sardis (about 400) recounts how Plotinus, one of the most gifted of the Neo-Platonic school, repeatedly proved himself to be a medical miracle-worker, most conspicuously during the sickness of Porphyrius. When the latter, a favorite disciple of Plotinus, was traveling through Sicily he became dangerously ill—in fact, according to the description of Eunapius, he was actually breathing his last. Then Plotinus appeared, and by magic words cured the dying man instantly. It appears, moreover, that Plotinus did not only operate with wonder-working words, but he employed still other agencies—as, for instance, mysterious figures (ὀχήματα. Villoison, Anecd. græca, Vol. II., page 231). Plotinus was even said to possess his own demon, who was at his disposal alone, and by the aid of whom he performed other wonders—as, for instance, that of prophesying.

Porphyrius, probably the most notable disciple of the Neo-Platonic school after Plotinus, claimed even that the demons personally taught him to expel, with certainty and despatch, those pathogenic demons. It was claimed by him that Chaldean and Hebrew words and songs were the promptest means of turning out all these evil spirits; in fact, the philosopher, Alexander of Abonoteichos, in Paphlagonia, was of the opinion that a pestilence, which was devastating Italy, could not be checked by any better means than that of affixing to the doors of the infected towns and villages the sentence: "Phœbus, the hair unshorn, dispels the clouds of disease."

Thus the last great system into which the ancient philosophy developed was attended by the unfortunate result of a very material increase of superstition in the healing art. This recrudescence of medical superstition was by no means a transitory one, but proved exceedingly persistent; in fact, we may unhesitatingly maintain that from that time superstition never again disappeared from our science. This is principally the fault of the position which Christianity took with regard to demonology and the other fantastic ideas of Neo-Platonism.

Early Christianity, from the outset, was subjected to the influence of ancient false ideas on the subject of demons. Without making any modifications whatever, it had appropriated this false doctrine, and had deduced from it the same medical notions as paganism had done. The New Testament exhibits numerous examples of a prevailing belief that supernatural beings—i.e., demons—were frequently the cause of bodily ailments; and as Christ and His disciples had often cured such patients, it follows that the belief in demons and their relations to pathology must have been widely disseminated among the Christians of that period. The Church Fathers also bear witness to this fact, as they, in their writings, acknowledge, in plain terms, the belief in demons as causes of disease. Justin Martyr, Tatian, Tertullian, Origen, Augustin, all mention demons and their power over the human body (compare Harnack, Chapter V., page 68, etc., where these conditions are most lucidly depicted). Thus, for instance, St. Augustine says: *"Accipiunt (scilicet dæmones) enim sæpe potestatem et morbos immittere et ipsum aerem vitiando morbidum reddere."*

And, indeed, early Christianity not only accepted pagan demonology unchanged, it even increased the therapeutic aspect of this delusion in a most regrettable manner. This belief in demons, under the influence of Christian doctrines, developed into an epidemic of insanity which prevailed unrestrictedly for two or three centuries, and which was again awakened in the late middle ages, to grow at last into one of the most terrible aberrations of the human mind—into the belief in witches.

This epidemic derangement of the mind, to which the belief in demons tended, under the influence of Christian doctrines, culminated in the patient's manifest idea that he was possessed of a demon. The mental disturbance set in with wild, spasmodic attacks of excitement, and, as it occurred not only in individual cases, but was also contagious, we must not hesitate to designate this belief of the first three centuries in demoniac possession an epidemic disease. It was an affection, the mental substratum of which consisted in a mixture of overheated religious sentiment and unrestrained medical superstition. The extent to which this belief in demoniac possession was disseminated during the first centuries of the Christian era is shown by the fact that a number of persons busied themselves with the cure of this affection. In the first place, most Christian communities owned an exorcist, or official caster-out of demons. It seems that this profession of exorcists formed a clerical order of its own; for, as all pagans, according to the Christian conception, were in the power of evil spirits, these demons were to be thoroughly driven out before each baptism, and thus the institution of a special church officer, whose duty it was to drive out demons, became absolutely necessary, especially after exorcism had also been introduced, during the fourth century, in the baptism of children. It may be stated, incidentally, that Catholic clergy of the third minor order are even to-day called "exorcists."

The Christian exorcists, in conjuring, only made use of prayer and of the name of Christ; these two factors were considered sufficient to cure the patient of his delusions, and they actually did so. Why they accomplished a cure has been explained very strikingly by Harnack. He says: "It is not the prayer that cures, but the praying person; not the formula, but the spirit; not exorcism, but the exorcist. Only in those cases in which the disease, as in numerous cases of the second century, had become epidemic and almost common, did ordinary and conventional means avail. The exorcist became a mesmerizer, possibly a deceived deceiver. But when strong individuality is deceived concerning its own personality by the demon of terror, and the soul is actually shaken by the power of darkness which possesses it, and from which it purposes to escape, a powerful and holy will alone can interfere from the outside world to deliver the shackled will. In some cases we find traces of a phenomenon which in modern times, for want of some better name, has been called 'suggestion'; but the prophet suggests in a different manner than does the professional exorcist."

Besides these official Christian exorcists, a great multitude of other persons carried on the trade of conjurer of demons. The sorcerers and magicians who plied their nefarious trade for the cure of the possessed and for those suffering from other diseases, worked with various kinds of mystic signs and ceremonies, and they certainly did an excellent business, for he who humors the superstition and the stupidity of man always prospers. Modern quackery illustrates this most strikingly. But, besides these healers, there existed numerous other conjurers of demons and medical wonder-workers who plied their trade not for the sake of contemptible mammon, but solely for ethical reasons. These were the members of the various theosophico-philosophical sects, who were active during the first Christian centuries and have been exhaustively described on the previous pages.

Altho Christians were eager to exalt their exorcists, who worked only with prayer and the invocation of Christ, above all practises of sorcery, they were not able, in the long run, to prevent Christian dogmas from being confounded with and corrupted by those of philosophy. Under the influence of Saturninus, Basilides, and Carpocrates, the various philosophical vagaries concerning accessory, intermediary, and inferior gods, and their influences upon the fate of man, corrupted the pure and simple teachings of Christ. That error against which Paul had so impressively cautioned the early Christian communities in his Epistle to the Colossians, Chapter II., verse 8 ("Beware lest any man spoil you through philosophy and vain deceit, after the tradition of men, after the rudiments of the world, and not after Christ"), had, nevertheless, made its appearance at last, and the adulteration of pure Gospel by philosophical speculations and fantastic views began to grow more complete from the third century on. This was the foundation of the religio-mystic system which, during the middle ages, and even beyond the period of the Renaissance, oppressed humanity like a suffocating nightmare, and not only checked progress, but also filled each branch of human knowledge with the most frightful superstition and the crassest mysticism. This was the case also in medicine; in fact, this branch of science has probably suffered most from the alliance of Christianity with the fantastic doctrines of philosophical schools.

The ancient doctrine of demons passed under the influence of Christian mysticism through certain changes and transitions, especially in its relation to the bodily condition of individuals. The variations in this doctrine were naturally most plainly evidenced in the medical views of the day. It was believed that every human being from birth was allotted a good and an evil demon. The good spirit held his hand protectingly over his human charge, whereas the evil demon only waited his chance to inflict injury upon man, forming especially the determining principle in the etiology of disease. It is true, the evil spirits apparently were no longer allowed to have such full sway over the health of humanity as they formerly had. God now utilized them principally as executors of punishments which he intended for mankind as a retribution for various forms of delinquency. Thus the Church Father, Anastasius (Sprengel, Vol. II., page 210), tells us that the reason why so many lepers and cripples were found among Christians was that God, enraged at the luxury of the members of the community, had sent the evil demon of disease among them. The wrath of God from that time until late in modern times has been considered a fully efficacious principle of pathology; in fact, there are numbers of people even to-day who believe that not natural, but supernatural and unearthly, factors are active in the bodily ailments of mankind.

The idea of good and evil demons, however, now assumed a specifically Christian character which, it is true, greatly resembled the ancient Babylonian notion, excepting that the good demons were replaced by angels and saints, whereas the evil spirits were embodied in the devil. Both, saints as well as devils, were thenceforth destined to play a part in the domain of medicine. It is true, the general recognition which they enjoyed during the middle ages and a considerable period of modern times has probably now passed away, but there still exist numerous classes of our people in whom the medical rôle of saints as well as devils is most willingly acknowledged.

We have referred elsewhere to the therapeutic accomplishments of the saints during the middle ages. We will here only dwell upon the influence which the devil, the Christian successor of the ancient evil spirit, has exerted upon the medical views of all classes of the people. This influence was very great. The devil and his subordinate infernal spirits were considered the "disturbers of peace" in the health of humanity. Disease in its various forms was their work; they resolved to inflict it either from inherent villainy or as incited by various magical arts of evil men. It was especially the latter form of diabolical activity that, during the entire middle ages and during a considerable part of modern times, was accepted as uncontestedly authentic, and the imagination of mankind at that period was inexhaustible in inventing the greatest variety of infamous actions which the devil was able to perform either of his own accord or as summoned by incantations. Any one desiring to acquaint himself thoroughly with these delusive ideas should read the work of the Friar Cæsarius, who lived about 1225, in the Rhenish-Cistercian monastery of Heisterbach. Naturally, we are only interested in the medical acts which the devil was always ready to perform. According to the history of medical superstition, the devil, who was invoked by various spells or appeared of his own volition, was able to influence each individual bodily organ in a manner most disagreeable to the possessor of the same. Neither were the Prince of Hell and his hosts always satisfied to tease and to plague an individual being, but very frequently they carried on this business wholesale. They threw themselves upon the entire population of a country, and caused sickness in all who crossed their path. The great epidemic of St. Vitus's dance of the fourteenth century, for instance, was considered to be the work of the devil, and the clergy busied themselves in driving out this devil's pest by means of sprinkling holy water and by the utterance of conjuring formulas.

The sexual life of men as well as of women offered an especially fruitful field for the activity of the devil and of his infernal companions. Thus, it was a favorite trick of the ruler of hell and of his subordinate demons to assume the shape of the husband or lover of this or that female, and, under this mask, to assume rights which should be permitted only to the husband. The infernal spirit that played this rôle was called Incubus. Thus, for instance, Hinkmer tells us of a nun who was mischievously claimed by such an infernal paramour, and who could be relieved of him only by priestly aid. But hell also contained female constituents who played the same rôle for the male as did Incubus for women. Such a wanton woman of hell was called Striga or Lamia (compare Hansen, pages 14 and 72). These amorous female friends of hell did not even stop when they met eminent saints. In the convent of St. Benedetto, near the Italian town of Subiaco, a rose-bush is shown even to-day into which the naked St. Benedict threw himself in order to resist the unholy temptation. And every one is sufficiently acquainted with the troubles which St. Anthony of Padua had with these infernal women. However, we physicians know well enough the cause of these temptations. They may surely and actually have approached the nun of whom Hinkmer reports, also St. Benedict and St. Anthony; however, they were not the devil's prostitutes, but the expressions of suppressed and disregarded impulses of nature which, in the form of voluptuous imaginations, appeared before the eyes of persons removed from terrestrial gratifications; for nature does not even exempt a saint, and the ancient saying, *"Naturam expellas furcâ, tamen usque recurret,"* applies to them as well as to any other mortal.

Finally these liberties which the devil and his infernal host were said to take as regards matters pertaining to love, assumed general and quite serious forms; in fact, they gave rise to delicately contrived legal questions. Namely, the idea had suggested itself that the devil was able not only to call forth promiscuous love between men and women, but that sometimes he derived a particular enjoyment if he could manage to prevent a marriage that had already been consummated by rendering the husband impotent. *Maleficium* was the technical term for such an event, equally saddening to husband as to wife, and the theologians, philosophers, and jurists of the middle ages have written the most learned commentaries regarding the legal consequences of this *impotentia ex maleficio*. It was disputed whether or not this form of impotence would constitute a legal cause for dissolution of marriage which, after all, was a divine institution; the reasons also why God permitted the devil to play such a reprehensible game were investigated in a most serious and profound manner. Any one interested in this question of*impotentia ex maleficio* may read the most excellent description of this subject by Hansen (Chapter III.).

This *impotentia ex maleficio*—i.e., one of the most extravagant outgrowths of medical superstition— occasionally also gave rise to scandalous lawsuits. This was the case in the disgraceful divorce suit which took place about the year 860 between King Lothaire II. and his spouse Teutberga. Lothaire was said to have lost his procreative power completely, owing to infernal artifices of his concubine,

Waldrada. The reason why a concubine should undertake such a step, which, after all, was bound to discredit her title and office in the eyes of her lover, is not quite evident. However, at that period it was not difficult to find an explanation for this remarkable fact. It was stated, e.g., that Waldrada was instigated to this act solely by jealousy and selfishness, in order to divorce the king from his consort. This first step once taken, the courtesan, by removing the spells cast by her, would take good care that the king should soon be delivered from the odious condition of impotence. However, Waldrada had reckoned without her host— i.e., in this case, without Hinkmar, Archbishop of Rheims; for this latter gentleman, exceedingly well versed in all matters ecclesiastic, politic, and diabolic, a genuine clerical fighting-cock, very soon closely investigated the impotence of his royal master. In an extensive memorial he considered the royal impotence according to its legal, theologic, philosophic, moral, and various other aspects. Medical superstition, accordingly, had acquired such power that the sovereign of the holy Roman and German empires had to submit his *potestas in venere* to the test of public discussion.

But conditions were to become much worse. When, about the thirteenth century, scholasticism had usurped full control of human reason, and all sciences were permitted to be pursued only in a scholastic sense, medicine was entirely divorced from the actual conditions of life. It was completely detached from nature, its great teacher, and irretrievably entangled in the subtleties of an uncertain philosophy. Its activity now depended exclusively upon the study of the ancients—by no means, however, upon that study in which an attempt was made to master the intellectual spirit of ancient medicine, but which consisted in a slavish adherence to the letter. Every decision of the ancients, without any regard to nature, was made a dogma, and he was the best physician who was most familiar with these dogmas, who understood best how to interpret them most keenly. Mankind had entirely lost the conception that the ancients had attained worth and importance only in that they measured things by the standard of unbiased experience, and tested their conclusions according to the phenomena of nature as described from accurate observation of the sick.

It is quite obvious that superstition met with a well-prepared soil in a system of medicine that was overburdened with dogmas and degraded into utter subserviency to a vainglorious philosophy. The natural result was that the medical art of a period of the middle ages, steeped in scholasticism, was nothing but a chaos of the most despicable superstition and folly. The most shocking result of these conditions was the belief in witches, and, with this, medical superstition entered upon a new stage. Whereas until then it had possessed a restricted, mere local vitality, and entailed danger only upon those who, from thoughtlessness, lent a willing ear to it, now it degenerated into a mental epidemic which threatened equally all classes of the people. The unspeakable misery which this variety of medical superstition has brought to the Western world is well known, so that we may refrain from entering into details, referring our readers to the excellent work of Hansen on this subject.

Physico-medical thought was so thoroughly destroyed by the above-described conditions that, even when humanity commenced to shake off the scholastic yoke, during the period of Renaissance, medicine was only able, in part, to follow this lead. Altho, under the inspiration of the ancients, it returned to nature, it was not able to rid itself of the superstitious idea of the continuous interference of supernatural powers with the performance of the most common functions of the body. The Church still persisted in the implicit belief in such views, and still dominated men's minds so thoroughly that even many physicians, who in other respects were entirely unbiased, remained on this point dutiful children of the Church; in fact, even those who were fully aware of the shortcomings of the Christian Church unhesitatingly adhered to the belief in demons as developed from antique conceptions by the Church Fathers. Thus, for instance, Dr. Martin Luther was a strict believer in the doctrine which taught men to hold the devil responsible for the origin of all diseases. He thus expressed himself, for instance: "No disease comes from God, who is good and does good to everybody; but it is brought on by the devil, who causes and performs all mischief, who interferes with all play and all arts, who brings into existence pestilence, Frenchmen, fever, etc." He accordingly believed that he himself was compelled to scuffle with the devil when his physical condition was out of order. Thus, when suffering from violent headache, he wrote to the Elector, John of Saxony: "My head is still slightly subject to him who is the enemy of health and of all that is good; he sometimes rides through my brain, so that I am not able to read or to write," and upon another occasion he said, in regard to his health: "I believe that my diseases are by no means due to natural causes, but that 'Younker Satan' plays his pranks with me by sorcery."

The devil was also held responsible for the appearance of monsters; it was believed that the ruler of hell helped young girls against their will to enjoy the delights of motherhood. However, these delights were said to be of a peculiar kind, in that intercourse with the devil was always bound to be followed by the birth of the most frightful monsters. The devil then unloaded these most remarkable monsters into respectable people's houses. Even Luther was not able to free himself from this most astonishing delusion. On the contrary, he was devoted to it with such conviction that, when once in Dessau, he heard of a monster (according to medical opinion, it was a question of a rhachitic child) that had grown to be twelve years of age, he advised, in all seriousness, that this sinful product of devilish intercourse be thrown into the river Mulde (compare Möhsen, Vol. II., page 506, etc., on "The Relations of Luther to the Devil").

If it was very improper of the devil to visit even clerical gentlemen, he crowned his wickedness, in that he very unceremoniously honored even ministers in the pulpit with his visit. Such an occurrence took place in Friedeberg, Neumark, in 1593, in which otherwise harmless town the devil commenced suddenly to create an unheard-of commotion. He harassed about one hundred and fifty people, and even in church he gave so little rest to those he possessed, that they raised various kinds of mischief in this holy place. When, thereupon, the preacher, Heinrich Lemrich, thundered against these deviltries from the pulpit, the devil became so incensed that immediately he promenaded into the Reverend Lemrich himself, so that the good minister raged in the pulpit exactly as did the members of his congregation down below in the nave.

However, this variety of medical superstition finally spread to such an extent that, as medical aid was powerless against the devil, the aid of God, by order of the consistory, was invoked from all pulpits of the Margravate against the above-described misdeeds of hell's ruler.

But the clergy adopted still another plan to checkmate the devil. In various publications they enumerated the villainies which Satan might visit on mankind, so that each and every one would be enabled to protect himself against the aggressions of the devil, in whatever form he might make his appearance. The first publication of this character was issued in 1555 by the General Superintendent of the Electorate of Brandenburg, Professor of the University of Frankfort, Herr Musculus; it bore the very appropriate title, *The Pantaloon Devil*. In fact, as early as 1575 a compilation was published in Frankfort-on-the-Main, in which twenty-four different forms, which the devil might assume in visiting humanity, were discussed most conscientiously and with becoming diffuseness of style (compare Möhsen, Vol. II., page 426, etc.).

From that time it was impossible for mankind to shake off the belief in devil and demons. The thought of being possessed played a conspicuous part even in the first half of the nineteenth century, thanks to the activity of Justinus Kerner, and even medicine felt called upon to busy itself more thoroughly with this newly resurrected belief. This was done, for instance, by Dr. Klencke, who, in 1840, published a little book exclusively for the purpose of disproving the existence of spirits.

We have so far shown the potent influence exerted upon medical superstition by antique as well as by medieval philosophy. But the newer philosophy greatly influenced the destiny of medicine, even at the end of the eighteenth and at the beginning of the nineteenth centuries. The natural philosophy based upon the doctrines of Schelling once more submerged the art of healing in mysticism, and thus necessarily abetted superstition. The physician no longer conceived disease as the effect of disturbances in the life of the bodily organs, but held various forms of inconceivable powers responsible for the incidence of a malady. The soul wrapped in sin had power to lead the life of the body from the normal into the pathological condition, and, accordingly, prayer and the belief in Christian dogmas again became active as curative factors. It was especially the Munich clinician, Nepomuk von Ringseis, who placed such theories before his pupils, and who, in his "System of

Medicine," published in 1840, made them generally known. Ringseis states in this book: "As disease is originally the consequence of sin, it is, altho not always indispensable, yet according to experience, incomparably more safe that physician as well as patient should obtain absolution before any attempt at healing be made." Another passage reads: "Christ is the all-restorer, and as such He cooperates in every corporeal cure." In this sense Ringseis calls the sacraments "the talismans coming from the Physician of all physicians, and, therefore, the most excellent of all physical, stimulating, and alterative remedies."

Thus, after almost three thousand years, medicine had returned to the stage at which it originated—namely, to the view that incorporeal, supernatural factors were to play a determining part in pathology and therapy. However, that there are plenty of individuals even in our time who are at any moment ready again to sacrifice wantonly all enlightenment and all progress to this varied superstition, is demonstrated by the cases of Mrs. Eddy and the Reverend Dowie, those modern representatives of medical superstition. There is only one protection against these relapses, against these atavistic tendencies, and that is education in natural science. The more it becomes disseminated among the people the less danger there will be that the heresies of a false philosophy, or of an overheated religious sentiment, may again conjure up medical superstition to the detriment of humanity.

V

THE RELATIONS OF NATURAL SCIENCE TO MEDICAL SUPERSTITION

THE point of view from which man has regarded nature for thousands of years up to modern times has been such as to promote most effectually the development of superstition; for the idea that a satisfactory insight into the character of natural phenomena can be obtained only by means of adequate experiments, and of observation perfected by the employment of the inductive reasoning and ingenious instruments, is comparatively recent. Natural science applying such means is scarcely two hundred years old. Fit instruments for the observation of nature existed only to a limited extent up to the eighteenth century, and, besides, their complete efficiency left much to be desired. The attempts to wrest from Nature her secrets by means of experiment were but feeble and unsuccessful. Altho the ancients, as is shown by the writings of Hippocrates, Galen, and others, had some knowledge of vivisection, they had practised it to a most limited extent. During the middle ages and the period of the Renaissance comparatively few physical experiments were made. Whatever researches in natural science were then undertaken were intended much less for the investigation of nature than for fantastic and superstitious purposes—as, for instance, the investigations of alchemy and astrology.

It is quite obvious that, under such circumstances, a number of superficial, imperfect, and distorted observations crept into the theoretic system of natural science.

However, this was not all; the diagnostico-theoretical method, by means of which antiquity, the middle ages, and even the greatest part of more modern times, had seen the natural sciences treated, was radically wrong. Man did not feel his way carefully from experiment to experiment, from observation to observation, until the general principle was found which inductively comprised a number of phenomena under one uniform principle of law, but the principle which was at the bottom of phenomena was fixed upon a speculative basis, and in accordance with this principle the phenomena were interpreted— as was done, for instance, in medicine in the case of humoral pathology. And as this speculatively constructed principle was obtained exclusively by a method dangerous to the cognition of natural sciences, by conclusion from analogy, naturally the most fantastic and adventurous conceptions soon became accepted in the realm of natural philosophy. But natural philosophy once lost in such a labyrinth, an aberration of the perceptive powers can not fail to follow—at least, in certain domains of nature. As a matter of fact, this fallacious perception promptly made its appearance, and has proved the stumbling-block of science from its earliest days up to the present times. Occultism, mysticism, or whatever the names may be of the various forms of superstition, have sprung from these erroneous conceptions of natural science. It may even be contended that no variety of superstition exists which is not somehow connected with a distorted observation or explanation of nature. However interesting these considerations may be, we can not here pursue them any further.

Such investigations belong to the history of superstition in general, and any one who desires more detailed information is referred to the enormous literature of the subject. We can here consider only those relations which prevail, or have prevailed, between superstition and natural science, and principally the influence which was thus exerted upon the art of healing by astronomy.

Astronomy and medicine became most intimately connected during the earliest periods of human civilization. The literature of cuneiform inscriptions shows us that the attempt to bring the stars into connection with human destinies is primeval, and reaches back to the ancient Babylonian age, even to the Sumero-Accadic period (Sudhoff, *Med. Woche.* 1901, No. 41). How primeval peoples came to connect their destinies with the heavenly bodies and their orbits is explained so lucidly by Troels-Lund (page 28, etc.) that we shall cite his descriptions, even if they are rather long for quotation. He says: "The Chaldean history of creation is inscribed upon seven clay tablets. On the fifth tablet we read: 'The seventh day He instituted as a holy day, and ordained that man should rest from all labor.' Why just seven? Because the holy number seven of the planets imperceptibly shone through the work of creation, and was imperceptibly impressed upon the entire order of thought. We are here at the decisive epoch at which the planets for the first time gave an impetus to human conception, the effects of which were to persist for thousands of years. This was repeated a second time when Copernicus, in dealing especially with the orbit of the planets, founded the still-prevailing conception of the universe.

"For the theory of creation could be reconciled with the phenomenon of sun and moon moving in their regular courses. They were in this case no longer, as had been assumed until then, individual living beings and divinities, but lights kindled by a mighty God, and intended to move day and night, in an established order, under the dome of heaven. But the other five planets! It was unnecessary to be a Chaldean on the Babylonian Tower in order to feel amazement at these. Every one who had ever followed with his eye their courses for a few nights during a caravan journey, every one who, lying awake, had occasionally attempted to read the time from the only clock of the night—the star-covered canopy of heaven—was bound to have noticed their peculiarities as to light and course. They did not shine uniformly, but sometimes intensely, at other times faintly, and entirely different was their radiance from that of other stars—reddish, greenish, bluish. And their course was at one time rapid, at other times slow; then backward or oblique; sometimes they disappeared entirely. Necessarily they appeared inexplicable not only to the inexperienced observer, but to a still higher grade of intellect—that of the most experienced Chaldean; for, altho their periods could possibly be calculated, their courses beggared all geometrical figures. These confused paths could be explained only in one manner—namely, as the expression of an arbitrary will, the manifestations of an independent life. The courses of the planets furnished the astronomic proof that the heavenly bodies were animated. The universe was more than created, it was godhead itself in living activity.

"How this point of view broadened and cleared everything! The world assumed the shape of an enormous hall upon which divine power, divine will, continuously acted from above. Farthest down was the world of the elements. In boundless distances above it moved the moon and the six other planets, each one in its transparent heaven. In the highest height, finally, revolved the canopy of impervious heaven, into which constellations were ranged in shapes that resembled animals (Tablet V., verse 2). Apparently these rotations did not have anything in common with each other; a power which passed through them from above moved these elemental worlds. Did not daily experience of their rising determine winter, storm, drought, etc.? Thus the processes on earth only reflected and repeated the course of these divine and heavenly bodies; yea, divine will itself. But their order of movement varied. Sun and moon with their regular courses spin, as it were, the firm warps and woofs; the other five are instrumental in producing what is changeable and apparently accidental. Unitedly in their course through heaven the seven weave the threads of fate. Silently they weave the design of terrestrial life. Upon

115

them depend not only summer and winter, rain and drought, but also the life and death of every living being; as determined by the constellation of their birth, such is each man, so will he live. Never do the heavenly bodies repeat precisely the same relative positions, and, therefore, never are two years, two days, two human beings, two leaves, completely identical."

So far Troels-Lund.

Much as we agree with what Troels-Lund says, yet we believe that the decisive motive which led humanity to bring their bodily welfare into closest connection with the starry canopy of heaven was suggested by the powerful influence which the sun exerts upon the bodily welfare of all life. As this life-giving power of the sun had a conspicuous share in the origin of primeval sabianism, so also it exerted a similar influence upon the development of astrology; for it must have been obvious to even the most stupid observer that his well-being depended to a great extent upon the action of the sun. From this perception to the idea that other heavenly bodies were also intended to exert a decisive influence upon things terrestrial was only a short step for the ancient civilized peoples; for here the conclusion from analogy was actually so closely and so enticingly under every one's nose that all he had to do was but to pitch upon the powers which rule all earthly life and neatly box them up in a well-constructed system. But as the conclusion from analogy was always considered in the ancient world as the most certain, never-failing path to knowledge, it was readily followed in this connection also. And thus astrology, like the greater part of medico-physical knowledge, was based, we think, upon the treacherous ground of a conclusion *per analogiam*.

Besides, our opinion that the warming and vitalizing power of the sun formed one of the most important factors in the origin of astrology is confirmed by the utterances of astrologists themselves. Thus, for instance, Ptolemy points to the sun and moon as the sources of life to mankind, and Hermes and Almansor repeat the dictum. This is furthermore proved by the unparalleled popularity which astrology has enjoyed in all phases of civilization. There is no civilized people, either of ancient or of modern times, which has not adhered to astrologic doctrines with the fullest confidence and most unswerving faith. Babylonians, Egyptians, Greeks, Romans, Germans, Romanians—in short, all nations—have professed their belief in astrology. Such a conformity of opinion would, however, be inexplicable amid such a dissimilarity of religious and cultural ideas as characterized the different peoples, unless a common principle had decisively influenced all nations in the same manner. This principle was acknowledged in the influence of the sun. Every human being was bound to observe the animating power of the sun on his own bodily sense and from his own observation, and would be at once led to the conclusion that a similar power resided also in the other celestial bodies.

This conception, which to a great extent was brought about by conclusions from analogy, provided a method of inference concerning various other phenomena. Man meditated, speculated, concluded, until the required sidereal relation of each organ and each function of the human body was determined. Thus astrology may serve as one of the most telling examples of scientific delusions to which the ancient diagnostico-theoretical methods were bound to lead, with their conclusions from analogy and their deductive modes of procedure.

The above survey indicates, altho only in very general outlines, the origin of astrology. We shall now consider more in detail the acquisition for which the art of medicine is especially indebted to astrology.

Babylonico-Assyrian civilization possessed in its earliest ages a well-developed system of astrologic medicine, as is evident from writings bequeathed to us from antiquity. Campbell-Thompson has recently published, from the great stock of cuneiform tablets in the collection of the British Museum, 276 inscriptions of an astrological nature belonging to the so-called Kouyunjik collection. Sudhoff has compiled them, so far as they refer to medicine, and has subjected them to critical analysis. We take the liberty of repeating certain extracts from these cuneiform tablets, which appear to be the reports which Assyrian and Babylonian court astrologists made to the king.

Tablet 69a says: "If the wind comes from the west upon appearance of the moon, disease will prevail during this month."

Tablet 207: "If Venus approaches the constellation of Cancer, obedience and prosperity will be in the land ... the sick of the land will recover. Pregnant women will carry their confinements to a favorable termination."

Tablet 163: "If Mercury rises on the fifteenth day of the month, there will be many deaths. If the constellation of Cancer becomes obscured, a fatal demon will possess the land and many deaths will occur."

Tablet 232: "If Mercury comes in conjunction with Mars, there will follow fatalities among horses."

Tablet 175: "If a planet becomes pale in opposition to the moon, or if it enters into conjunction with it, many lions will die."

Tablet 195: "If Mars and Jupiter come in conjunction, many cattle will die."

Tablet 117: "If the greater halo surrounds the moon, ruin will be visited upon mankind."

Tablet 269: "If an eclipse of the sun occurs on the twenty-ninth day of the month of Jypar, there will be many deaths on the first day."

Tablet 271: "An eclipse at the morning watch causes disease.... If an eclipse takes place during the morning watch, and lasts throughout the watch, while the wind blows from the north, the sick in Akkad will recover."

Tablet 79: "If a halo surrounds the moon and if Regulus stands within, women will bear male children."

Tablet 94: "If sun and moon ... on the fifteenth day 'answer my prayer' shall he say ... Let him nestle close to his wife, she shall conceive a son."

These few extracts show us the close relations into which Assyrico-Babylonian culture brought the becoming and passing away of all animal life with the stellar movement; in fact, as we note from Tablet 94, the astrologists of this period did not hesitate to intrude into the most intimate occurrences of married life. It is quite obvious that, under such circumstances, the Babylonian physician was compelled to consider very carefully the utterances of the astrologists in carrying on his practise. It may be possible that we shall obtain still further information regarding the quality of sidereal therapy from the numerously discovered cuneiform tablets. We know positively that a physician was forbidden to perform any surgical operations on certain days of each month. Thus, for instance, the 7th, 14th, 19th, 21st, and 28th of the month Schall-Elul were unfavorable days for such operations (Oefele). These directions were especially stringent in regard to venesection, to which act we shall again refer in greater detail.

When civilization, later on, continued to thrive upon the shores of the Nile, astrology still found a fertile soil there, and it appears that here also the name Ἰατρομαθηματικοί has originated, which, subsequently, was a favorite designation of adherents to the sidereal art of healing. The astrological prognoses made by the professional astrologist, Petosiris, for the king Nechepso of Sais are well known. However, it appears, according to the latest investigations (compare the excellent work of Sudhoff, page 4, etc.), that these prognoses have nothing at all to do with that king Nechepso who reigned in the seventh century, B.C. It seems more probable that some cunning Alexandrian astrologist of the second century,B.C., fraudulently used the name of the king as a cover for his work. But however this may be, these prognoses of Petosiris have considerable value, in that they give us an insight into the manufacture of such medical prophesies.

The object of these prognoses was primarily to discover the termination of a disease, whether the patient would die or recover, either soon or only after the lapse of a certain time—for instance, after seven days. This was all that Petosiris undertook to predict. All details regarding treatment, complications, and diagnosis of a case are still entirely wanting. Petosiris, in making such a prognosis, by no means relied solely upon the conjunction of certain celestial bodies, but he employed a rather intricate method, in which mystic numbers, onomancy, and astrology were important elements. To prognosticate medically according to this system a circle of numerals was required in the first place. There existed two different kinds of such circles—one simple, the other more complicated. Berthelot has furnished us with examples of both as used by Petosiris.

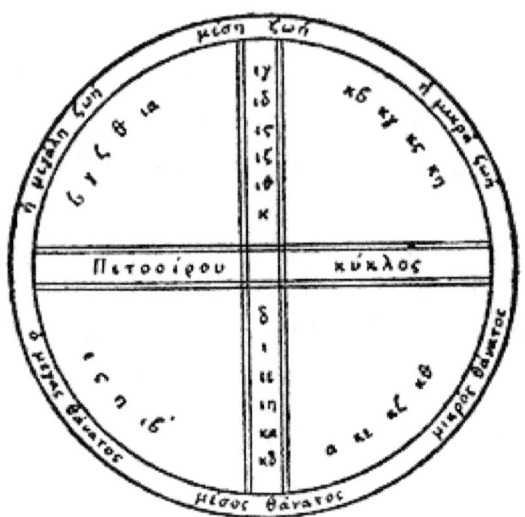

FIG. 1—CIRCLE OF PETOSIRIS
(After Bouché-Leclercq, p. 539)

The more simple formula (Fig. 1) consisted of two concentric circles, the smaller of which was divided into four quadrants. Between both concentric circles and within the horizontal diameters were inscribed the words: μέον ζωή; to the right of this: ἡ μικρὰ ζωή; to the left of the vertical line: ἡ μεναλη ζωή. Under the vertical line was inscribed: μέσος θάνατος; to the right of this: μικρὸς θάνατος; and to the left of the vertical line: ὁ μένας θάνατος. Only words which point to the longer or shorter duration of life, or to the death-struggle, were therefore employed. The four quadrants of the enclosed circle, as well as the vertical diameter, contained the numerals from 1 to 29 in a mystical order, representing the duration of the moon's phases. The above (Fig. 1) shows us this astrological circle of Petosiris.

The second—essentially more complicated—formula consists of three concentric circles. Various words are inscribed between the first and second circles, as in Fig. 1. Between the second and third circles, and in the verticals, the numerals from 1 to 30 are disposed in a mystical arrangement. Furthermore, these circles are not, as in Fig. 1, divided into four quadrants, but into eight equal sections. At these points in which the radii forming the sectors intersect the periphery of the outermost of the three concentric circles, arched enclosures are raised which also contain various words.

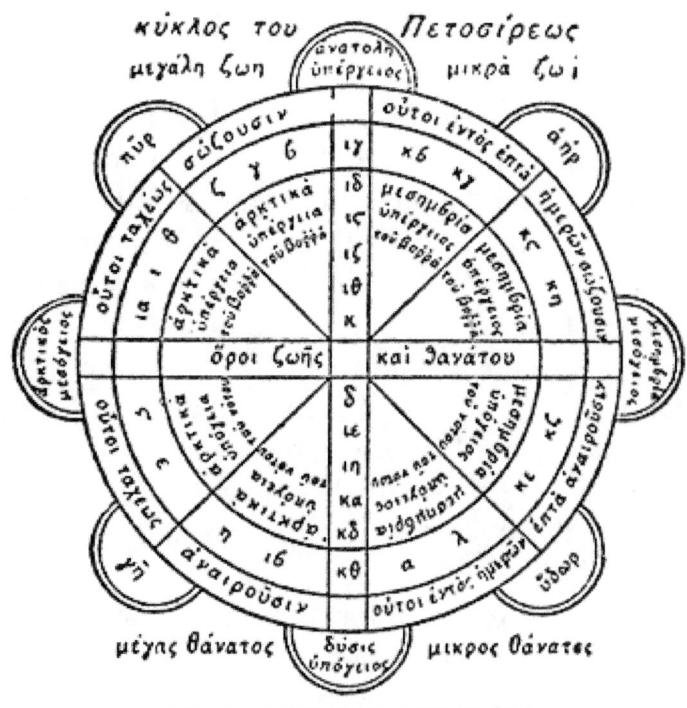

FIG. 2—CIRCLE OF PETOSIRIS
(After Bouché-Leclercq, p. 540)

When it was sought, by means of the above-described figures, to determine the medical future or the life and death of an individual, this could be accomplished with the aid of the diagram represented in Fig.1 in such a manner that the duration of the disease in days, the numerical value of the name of the patient, and the phases of the moon were added, and the sum divided by 29. The result thus obtained wasinterpreted by referring to the diagram. If this figure happened to be, for instance, in the right upper quadrant, the patient, altho he would recover from his illness, would live only for a very short period; if this number was found in the vertical line, below the horizontal diameter, the patient was destined to die after a short struggle.

Much more intricate was the use of the astrological apparatus illustrated in Fig 2. Here the number of the moon's day, and the numerical values of the name of the patient were not added, but each of these figures was separately looked for in the diagram. If the moon figure was found in the lower, the figure for the name in the upper, ends of the verticals—i.e., where δυσις ὑπόγειος, setting, and ἀνατολὴ ὑπέργειος, rising, stand—the individual concerned, altho in danger, finally recovered. If, on the other hand, the moon figure was discovered in the upper, and the figure for the name in the lower, ends of the verticals, nothing but evil was in store for the questioner, but the misfortune appeared under the guise of fortune. If both numbers, however, were at the upper ends of the verticals, the prospects were favorable, but bad if both figures occurred below the horizontal line.

A method which is similar to the simple apparatus of Petosiris is revealed to us in the so-called οφαῖρα Δημοκρίτου. It is contained in the *Papyrus Magica Musei Lugdunensis Batavia*, published by Dietrich. Fig. 3 shows the illustration belonging to this method, and also the Greek directions for use, as given in the papyrus. It will be noticed that in the method of Democritus recourse is made to a table of numerals divided by a cross-line into the upper and larger, and a lower and smaller, section. The upper part contains in three vertical columns 18, in the lower, 12 figures. To use the table, the day when the disease began, the numerical value of the name, and the days of the moon were added, and the sum thus obtained divided by 30. This quotient was then looked for in the table of numbers. If it was found above the cross-line, the patient recovered; if below, he succumbed.

α	ι	ιθ
β	ια	κ
γ	ιγ	κγ
δ	ιδ	κε
ζ	ιϛ	κϛ
θ	ιζ	κζ
ε	ιε	κβ
ϛ	ιη	κη
η	κα	κθ
ιβ	κδ	λ

FIG. 3—THE TABLE OF DEMOCRITUS

There existed a great many other methods besides those described above; for instance, the system of the 12 places, the circle of Manilius, the method of the mysterious Hermes Trismegistus, the circle of

Ptolemy, etc. However, we can not here enter into a more detailed description of these forms, and refer those that wish more exhaustive information to Berthelot, and, above all, to Bouché-Leclercq. Astrology, and, with it, sidereal medicine, subsequently traveled from its Oriental home into all civilized countries of the then known world.

As regards Greek and Roman antiquity, astrology in all its forms won a high reputation both in Greece and Italy. Even the most eminent ancient physicians, altho they did not unreservedly adopt sidereal medicine, refrained from disavowing it. Thus we find in the Corpus Hippocraticum, the chief work of early Greek medicine, passages which betray more than a friendly feeling toward the astral art of healing. It is true, expressions are not wanting which sound like a direct disowning of astrology.

Let us consider for a few moments the attitude of Hippocratic medicine toward astrology.

As to the rejection of astrologic medicine by the followers of Hippocrates, we read ("Ancient Medicine," Chapter I.; in the translation of Fuchs, Vol. I., page 19): "For this reason I believe that it [medical art] requires no basis of vain presumption, such as the existence of invisible and doubtful factors, the discussion of which, if it should be attempted, necessitates a hypothetic science of supernatural or of subterrestrial nature; for, if any one should contend that he knew anything about such a matter, neither he, the lecturer, nor his hearers would clearly understand whether his statements were true or not, because nothing exists to which reference could be had for purposes of verification."

This surely is a refutation as definite as can be desired of a medicine which depends upon witchcraft or astrologic vagaries. However, various other passages of the Corpus Hippocraticum take an exactly contrary position. For example, we find the following statement (on "Air, Water, and Locality," ChapterXVII., in the translation of Fuchs, Vol. I., page 390): "Attention must be paid to the rise of the stars, especially to that of Sirius,[4] as well as to the rise of Arcturus, and, further, to the setting of the Pleiades, for most diseases reach a crisis during such periods, some of them abating in these days, others ceasing entirely, or developing into other symptoms and different conditions." These words indicate a distinct intention of bringing prognosis and course of diseases into the closest relations with the motions of the celestial bodies. In the second chapter of the same book similar expressions occur: "He who knows how the change of seasons and the rising and setting of stars take place will also be able to foresee how the year is going to be. Therefore, any one who investigates these subjects and predicts coming events will be thoroughly informed as to each detail of the future; he will enjoy the best of health, and take as much as possible the right road in art. However, if any one should be of the opinion that these questions

---

[4] This star, in particular, played a rôle in the astrologic prognosis of the Egyptians; in fact, in various systems it was made the starting-point of medical predictions; for instance, in the method of Hermes Trismegistus.

belong solely in the realm of astronomy, he will soon change his opinion as he learns that astronomy is not of slight, but of a very essential, importance in medical art." Stars and diseases are also brought into mutual relations in the letter to King Ptolemy (Emerins, page 293).

The above quotations refer exclusively to the course of diseases in relation to the stars, but we find in other passages also distinct references are made to therapeutic methods; for instance, in "Aphorisms," § 4, paragraph 5, we read: "Purging is very difficult during or before the dog-days."

It would, indeed, be most remarkable if no astrologic remarks of any kind were found in the Corpus Hippocraticum, as the idea of close relation between the celestial bodies and matters terrestrial had common currency during the Hippocratic period. The songs of Stesichorus and of Pindar show, for instance (as is also stated by Pliny, Book 3, Chapter XII., Vol. I., page 118), that eclipses of certain stars were considered to be pregnant with mischief. This superstitious conception has, in some cases, actually caused severe general calamities. Thus, for instance, the Sicilian campaign ended unfortunately for the Athenians only because their general, Nicias, under a superstitious apprehension concerning an eclipse, failed to put to sea. And as this campaign was the cause to Athens of a partial loss of Greek hegemony, we may safely say that astrology had a decisive share in the fall of Athens (Pliny, Book 2, ChapterXXIII.).

The appearance of comets, like eclipses of the sun and the moon, were also reputed to be ominous among the ancients. Comets were considered heavenly mischief-makers of the worst kind, and almost every sort of calamity was ascribed to them. A calamity was supposed to assume various aspects, according to the position and form of the comet. Under some circumstances, however, they were said to prognosticate many events advantageous to mankind (Pliny, Book 2, Chapter XXIV.). Thus Augustus considered a comet, which was seen for an entire week at the northern quarter of the heavens at the onset of his rule, during performances which were given in honor of Venus genetrix, to be his lucky star.

However, not only such extraordinary appearances in the sky as comets, eclipses of the sun and the moon, played a conspicuous part in medical superstitions of the ancients. Even those celestial phenomena which occur with a regularity fixed by natural law, such as the revolution of the sun and the moon, were considered highly important events in therapeutic art. Thus, affections of the eye in man and beast were said to increase and to decrease with the moon (Pliny, Book 2, Chapter XLI.).

All acute diseases were believed to be controlled by the moon, whereas chronic affections were thought to be under the influence of the sun. In fact, everything that happened to man was brought in immediate relationship with appearances in the canopy of heaven. Thus, for instance, it is stated by Marcus Manilius, the well-known author of an astronomical didactic poem dedicated to the Emperor Augustus:

"Omnis cum coelo fortunæ pendeat ordo."

In the thirteenth chapter of the second book the poet maintains that each part of the human body is subordinate to a distinct sign of the zodiac. Thus, for instance, the head to Aries, etc.

Altho the further development of Occidental as well as Oriental astrology drew its resources from the primeval Assyrian, Babylonian, and Egyptian doctrines, yet from the second century, A.D., the astronomic work of Ptolemy and the exhaustive description of antique medicine by Galen derive their inspiration from *Medicina Astrologica*. Whatever these two great masters were able to report of the dependence of the functions of the body upon celestial bodies was from then on, without further inspection and examination, acknowledged to be true by the great majority of physicians. Only occasionally this or that practitioner is bold enough to oppose the intrusion of astrologic vagaries into the art of healing; among these radicals was the philosophically trained physician, Sextus Empiricus, who lived about the year 193, A.D. However, this protest of brave Sextus, as well as all subsequent ones, scarcely had any influence upon the astrological development of medicine. Astrology could not be arrested on its road to the domination of the world, and until the seventeenth century it controlled the thought of physicians with the same invincible sway that it exercised over the mental life of all other professions and classes. Medico-astrological superstition had become legalized, and this in spite of the fact that

130

Galen himself at last expressed his distrust of the *Medicina Astrologica*, and at least endeavored to extenuate his part in its dissemination.

Let us now scrutinize more minutely the condition of *Medicina Astrologica* in the second century, A.D. The works of Ptolemy, the "Iatromathematica" of the mysterious Hermes Trismegistus, and the third book of Galen's writing on the "critical days" furnish sufficient material for outlining the medico-astrological system of that period.

In the first place, the method by which the authors of that period instilled their astrologic dotage into the minds of their contemporaries varied considerably. Either astrological remarks were here and there interspersed in a work on medical or on astronomical subjects, as was the case, for instance, in the "Opus Quadripartitum" of Ptolemy and also in Galen's book on the "critical days," or astrology was treated as a special science in the form of a connected system, as is done, for instance, in the "Iatromathematica" of Hermes Trismegistus. Such textbooks of astrology obtained publicity in large numbers from about the fourteenth century on. Whoever may be inclined to cast a glance into the learned work of Sudhoff will be astonished to observe the extent to which iathromathematics flourished in the second half of the middle ages and at the turning-point of the Renaissance. Still another form was to impart to the public their astrological doctrines in the form of short sentences. We find nothing in such works regarding the intricate calculations and methods by which endeavors were made to fathom the language of the stars, but astrological results were communicated in concise, aphoristic sentences. This was done in the "Centiloquium" of Ptolemy, a work which in a hundred brief sayings brings an epitome of astrological wisdom to market. The work enjoyed the highest esteem in the middle ages. Such a book, therefore, would correspond to that form of modern literary production, which, under the title "Method of acquiring this or that accomplishment within a short period," is advertised to us modern people in the daily press. Moreover, the "Centiloquium" of Ptolemy had many imitators. Such a work is found, for instance, in Arabic literature, and contains astrologic wisdom condensed into 150 brief sentences by the astrologer Almansor, who furnished the handbook upon request of his ruler; the Arabian, Bethem, has produced a similar work. We find analogous works appearing later in the middle ages. Eventually, the doctrines of astrology were put into neat rhymes; thus, for instance, Heinrich von Rantzau, who departed this life 1598 as governor of Schleswig-Holstein, celebrates in 100 well-turned verses the significance of the planets in relation to the physical and mental welfare of humanity. We shall again refer to this subject when considering astrology of the middle ages. The iatromathematic passages in the above-mentioned writings of Ptolemy, Hermes, and Galen furnished the foundation for all later astrologico-medical theories. For what the middle ages believed regarding the medical importance of the sidereal world, especially of the planets and the zodiac, was nothing but the immediate continuation, or elaboration, of the astrologic teachings of Ptolemy and other authors of the first Christian centuries.

In the first place, every portion of the human frame was placed under the influence of a certain celestial body.

The five planets already known to the ancients, as well as sun and moon, governed, according to Hermes, the following parts of the body:

The sun, the right eye.The moon, the left eye.Saturn, hearing.Jupiter, the brain.Mars, the blood.Venus, taste and smell.Mercury, tongue and gullet.

However, the influence which sun, moon, and the planets exercised upon the human body gradually became more intricate. It was no longer satisfactory to enumerate relations between the bodies of heaven and the human organs of such a general nature as given by the above table of Hermes. All parts and functions of the body were to be brought into the closest relations with the planets. Thus, for instance, the celebrated humanist, Marsilius Ficinus, the friend of the Medici (1433 to 1499), depicts most minutely in a book "On Life," which was much read in its time, the relations between the body and the planets. This was also done by Heinrich von Rantzau, in his "Tractus Astrologicus," which in its time was very celebrated. There we read regarding these conditions as follows:

SATURN governs the spleen, the bladder, the bones, the teeth, and, in part, the circulating juices of the body; causes the color of the skin of man to be dark yellowish; impedes or promotes growth; causes the eyes to be small, and prevents the growth of the beard.

JUPITER governs the lungs, the ribs, cartilages, the liver, arteries, the pulse, and the development of human semen; causes the white color of the skin, and gives a good figure.

MARS governs the bile, kidneys, veins, and sexual organs, and of these especially the testicles; makes hair red and the temper irascible, and inclined to outrages of various kinds.

VENUS governs the uterus, the breasts, the sexual organs, the spermatic tubes, the loins, and the buttocks; endows man with physical beauty, furnishes him with long hair, round eyes, and a well-formed face; but it is inexcusable on the part of this star that it presented mankind with gonorrhea.

MERCURY governs all mental processes—memory, imagination, the brain with its nerves, the hands, feet, and legs, the bones and the bile; causes man to be light-fingered.

THE SUN governs the brain, nerves, urine, the right eye of the male and the left one of the female, the optic nerves, and the entire right half of the body; gives a good complexion to man.

THE MOON governs the brain, mouth, belly, intestines, bladder, taste, the organs of reproduction, the left eye of the male, the right eye of the female, and the feminine liver, and the entire left half of the body.

The signs of the zodiac, like the planets, exert full control over the various parts of the body. Honest Bartisch, of Königsbrück (1535 to 1606), has given us in his "Eye-Service" an illustration of these relations. Fig. 4 is a reproduction of this plate of Bartisch.

The sun, moon, planets, and zodiac regulated not only the life of the various limbs of living man placed under their special care, but their activity commenced at that moment when the foundation was just about to be laid for the future bodily existence of a mortal— i.e., at the moment of conception. If, during this critical process, the respective bodies of the heavens were in an unfortunate conjunction, the members of the future being, the most primitive forms of which had just been founded, were bound to suffer. Naturally, however, only those parts of the body were affected by this destiny which were in the care of stars that happened to be in unpropitious conjunction at the time.

If the act of conception had passed without evil influence on those that were actively and passively participating in it, the product of that hour could by no means be sure that this or that planet would not maliciously thwart the ease and tranquillity of its embryonic and fetal life. For sun, moon, and the seven planets each governed one month of intra-uterine life, as is explained by Jacobus Forliviensis. Saturn reigns during the first month of pregnancy, Jupiter in the second, Mars in the third, the sun in the fourth, Venus in the fifth, Mercury in the sixth, the moon in the seventh; the eighth month is ruled again by Saturn, and this latter planet now shows itself to be so malicious that it immediately destroys all life born in the eighth month. Jupiter again takes control during the ninth month, and, as this star is fond of warmth and humidity, and, therefore, a friend of life in any form, no danger is to be feared for a fetus entering the world during this month. However, after the nine months of pregnancy have passed without evil interference by the planets, Mars once more is in command, and his influence helps in accomplishing a normal birth.

After the fetus had successfully passed all dangers which the planets could cause during the nine months of intra-uterine life, and after it had successfully matured, the hour of birth might, after all, be accompanied with other quite severe sidereal complications. For if any planet was in an unfavorable sign, or if the relations between the signs of the zodiac and the sun or the moon were not quite in their regular order, those members which were presided over by the respective stars were made to suffer. The correctcasting of the medical horoscope, therefore, required the most accurate knowledge of the minute of birth, with simultaneous occurrences in the canopy of heaven. Provident fathers, accordingly, were mindful of having an astrologer, during the hour of birth, in the room in which the confinement was to take place, so that he might be able to ascertain as accurately as possible the celestial occurrences which would determine the bodily welfare of the new-born, and to arrange them for the horoscope.

After the young mortal had safely arrived, and if a fortunate destiny had placed in his cradle a favorable medical horoscope, both for the hour during which the first material foundation had been laid for his life and also for the hour of his birth, he had overcome only a small part of the troubles which the starry world might be able to inflict on his bodily welfare. If the various signs of heaven appeared in unfavorable conjunction, or if the moon entered into any fatal relations with the signs of the zodiac, members of the body which were under the influence of the respective celestial bodies were still imperiled. These dangers might threaten not only one individual, but they were capable, eventually, even of calling down epidemics and pestilence upon all humanity. After any form of disease had taken hold of a person its course, treatment, and termination could be clearly read in the stars of heaven.

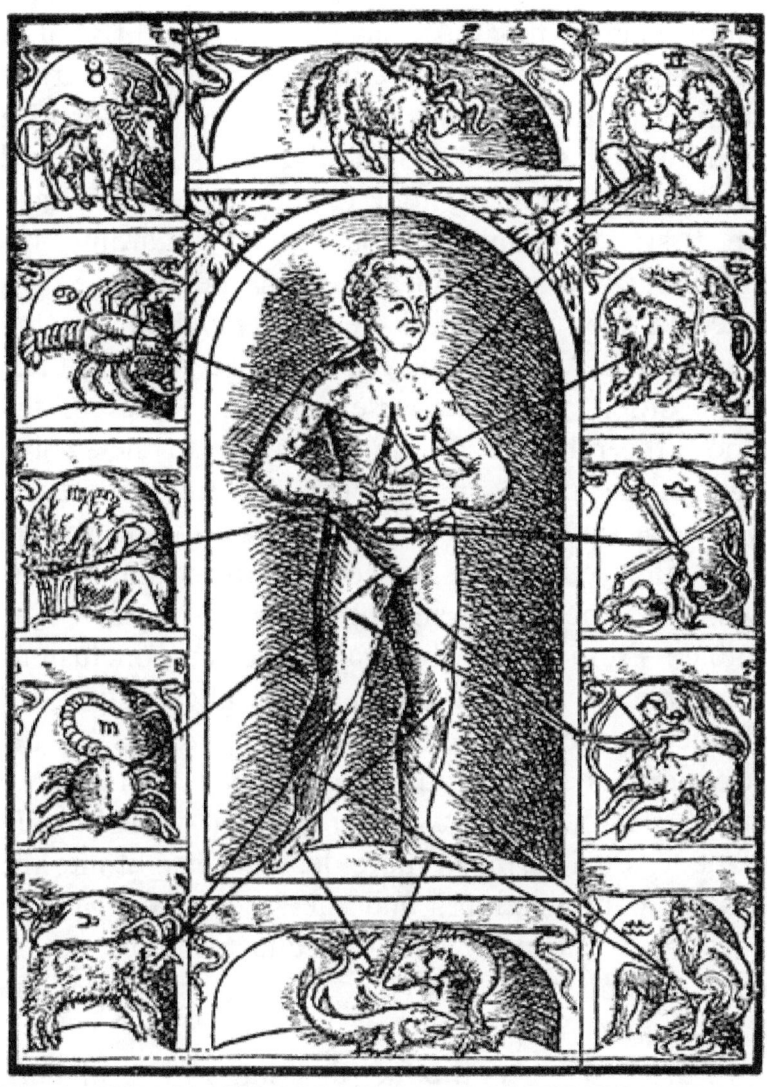

FIG. 4—THE RELATION OF THE PARTS OF THE HUMAN BODY TO THE SIGNS OF THE ZODIAC

It was necessary, above all, to ascertain the day, hour, and minute when the disease appeared. Unfortunately, this must have been quite difficult at times; for many diseases begin so insidiously that the moment of the attack is completely beyond precise definition. In such a case one did the best that could be done, and probably took as the moment of attack the first complaints of the patient regarding his disorder. After the appearance of the disease was dated in such a manner, the heavenly body, in the ascendant at this period, was then ascertained; thus, the position and the course and the phases of the moon, the relations of sun and moon to the twelve signs of the zodiac, and the planets would be noted. It was necessary to observe whether the moon was in opposition, quadrature, or conjunction to the planets while she stood in the sign of this or that figure of the zodiac. From these observations clear conclusions were first drawn regarding the general condition, the character, the duration, and the prognosis of the affection. These conclusions, however, were by no means satisfactory as yet. An attempt was therefore made to obtain a much more detailed insight into the causes, complications, and therapy of the case in question by means of astrology, and such information was abundantly provided in the *Medicina Astrologica*.

In the first place, the fact that sun, moon, planets, and the signs of the zodiac shared the rule over the various organs of the body, and furnished positive intimations regarding the cause of the disease in question, made it unnecessary for the physician to trouble himself at all with an examination of the patient in order to ascertain cause and localization of the affection. One glance at the conjunctions of the stars was sufficient to show which organ of the patient happened to be endangered by the celestial constellation. If an individual complained, for instance, of disturbed digestion, and if the heavenly body that presided over the liver presented any remarkable phenomena, naturally only the liver was responsible for the case in question, and the diagnosis was made. Complications were to be expected if the stars which controlled the circulation of blood and mucus showed unfavorable signs. It was even possible for the physician well versed in astrology to determine in advance the period of time at which the occurrence of such humoral complications might be expected, as he had learned that the various hours of the day and of the night were to exert a powerful influence upon the juices of the body. For instance, Almanzor explains that the first three hours of day and of night are in closest relation to the blood, whereas the second quarters of day and of night hold sway over the yellow, the third over the black (bile), and the last quarters, finally, over the mucus. However, not only were the various hours of great importance to the course of the disease, but certain days of the disease— so-called critical days—were of still greater significance. It is true, the doctrine of these critical days was by no means the property of *Medicina Astrologica*, but the Corpus Hippocraticum already contained a book Περὶ χρίησὶμων. But the followers of Hippocrates had developed this theory only from humoro-pathological premises, and Galen, in his work χρήίσιμαι ἡμέραι, had only included astrology in order to explain and to prove the entire doctrine of crises (compare also Sudhoff). He calculated in accordance with moon weeks and months, and in such a manner that a week counted six days and seventeen and one-half hours, and the month of the moon only twenty-six days and twenty-two hours. The seventh, fourteenth, twentieth, and twenty-seventh days were to be considered critical days of the first order. "Contemplate," says Galen, "the critical days in the course of the moon in the angles of a geometrical figure of sixteen sides; if you find these angles in a favorable constellation, the patient will fare well; badly, however, if evil signs prevail." But not only were certain hours and certain days of the week said to exert an important astrological influence upon the human body, such an influence was ascribed also to certain years. Such years were called *"Anni Scansiles"*—that is, "climacteric." The expression *"Anni Climacterici"* was also used, but this designation has nothing in common with the modern conception of the climacteric. It was believed that the condition of the body underwent a thorough revolution during these climacteric years, and that a new stage, as it were, of organic life was reached. Heinrich von Rantzau, the astronomic aristocrat and statesman, accordingly defines the climacteric years as *"anni, in quibus ad sequentis temporis constitutionem sese vertat ætas et inflectat."* Therefore, such years should in themselves harbor

140

dangers for corporeal existence, and offer no favorable prospect for the course of diseases.

Two kinds of such climacteric years were distinguished. One kind was brought about by multiplication with the figure 7, and they were called *anni hebdomatici,* or *climacterici (stricte sic dicta).* Accordingly, these were the years 7, 14, 21, 28, 35, 42, 49, 56, 63. These nine years formed the *climactericus parvus,* whereas the years 77, 84, 91, 98, 105, 112, 119, 126 were called the *climactericus magnus.* A multiplication which extended further, to 171, reached the *climactericus maximus.* The other kind of climacteric years was obtained by multiplication with 9, and such years were called *anni enneatici,* or*decretorii.* These were the years 9, 18, 27, 36, 45, 54, 63, 72, 81, 90, 99, 108, etc.

However, these climacteric years did not all present the same dangers, but the peril inherent in them varied considerably. It was determined by the multiplicator, and here especially the 3 and the 7 played a very fatal rôle. The 21st year of life (3 × 7), and the 27th (3 × 9), were one grade higher in the scale of dangers than those obtained by other multiplicators. Still more dangerous were those years arrived at by ascending in spaces of three hebdomads; therefore, the 21st year of life—i.e., the period of three hebdomads—namely, 3 × 7; the 42d year, as a period of 2 × 3 hebdomads— i.e., 2 × 21; the 63d year of life, as a period of 3 hebdomads—i.e., 3 × 21; 84 = to 4 × 21; 105 = 5 × 21, etc. The 49th year of life and the 56th year of life were said to be still more dangerous than these years obtained from the period of three hebdomads. It is true, the cause of the danger is quite obvious in the case of the 49th year; it was the ominous 7×7 which here gave rise to forebodings. And it was not quite comprehensible what caused the bad reputation of innocent 56; Rantzau fails to give us a sufficient explanation.

But the most dangerous climacteric year was the 63d, for this was made up of 7×9. It was, therefore, an *annus hebdomaticus* and, at the same time, also an *annus enneaticus*, for it belonged both to the class of those climacteric years which were formed by the multiplier 7, as also to that which were obtained by the multiplier 9. It was most natural, therefore, that a period of life which from two sides was fraught with danger, like the unfortunate 63d year of life, was bound to appear equally suspicious to the healthy and to the sick. It is probable that this year was, therefore, called *androdas*, because, as Rantzau believes, it debilitates and breaks vitality.

It would appear, moreover, that the climacteric years enjoyed general consideration in ancient times as well as in the middle ages, for Rantzau names a number of celebrated men who were said to have expressed themselves regarding the significance of these years, such as Plato, Censorinus, Gellius, Philo Judæus,Macrobius, Cicero,Boëtius, St. Ambrose, St. Augustine, Bede, Georgius Valla, and others. Not satisfied with this statement, Rantzau also mentions in his catalog a multitude of prominent men who all departed this life in their 63d year, and thus, as he believes, had established the dangerousness of this year by their death.

It is probable, therefore, that the 63d birthday was celebrated with great apprehension during the entire middle ages, and the respective individual did not draw an easy breath until after the ominous year had been successfully passed.

However, the stars knew not only how to tell particulars regarding the probable course and possible complications of diseases, but they also gave information regarding very special forms of affections. It was possible, thus, to learn from them at what time diseases of the eye were to be feared, when mental diseases were threatening, when hemorrhages were to be expected, etc. The astrologically trained physician was able to obtain prompt information from the stars regarding contingent surgical accidents; for there existed various conjunctions of the celestial bodies, according to Ptolemy, which surely pointed to wounds, fractures of bones, burns, concussions, and other lesions. In fact, it was possible to see in advance, from the celestial phenomena, what limbs would be exposed to forcible injury; thus, certain conjunctions of the planets were said to prognosticate with certainty wounds of the head; others, of the face; others, again, of the hands and feet, of the fingers and toes, of the arms and legs, of the trunk and neck. Astrology, moreover, was not satisfied with the prognostic and diagnostic activity which we have just mentioned, but it also interfered in therapy, internal as well as external.

Regarding, in the first place, internal medicinal treatment, the astrologer knew how to give positive information about the same; for all terrestrial beings, of an organic as well as of an inorganic nature, were under the influence of the sun, the moon, of the planets, and of the signs of the zodiac. The stars imparted certain powers to the planets, to animals, and to all structures of the inorganic world. If, therefore, it were known what stars happened to appear in the vault of heaven at the beginning of the disease or of its treatment, it was only necessary seriously to consider the organic and inorganic structures under their supervision, and the remedies required for a successful control of the disease were presently at hand. But if the healer wished to be absolutely certain what medicaments to choose, the phases of the moon and the condition of the sun were also to be taken into consideration. Some remedies could be administered only when the moon was in a particular relation to certain planets or stars of the zodiac. These remedies were principally emetics and purges.

Similarly to the internal clinician, so also in surgery, the healer was entirely dependent upon the conjunction of the stars. The primeval Babylonian directed that the body must not be touched with iron during certain conjunctions of the stars, and this was also prescribed in all cases of *Astrologica Medica*. It appears, however, that this direction obtained less general surgical recognition, but referred principally to blood-letting. Even to this limited extent it implied a high-handed interference with the art of the ancient as well as of the medieval physician; for venesection occupied an entirely different position among therapeutic measures during that period than it does to-day. Whereas modern medicine does not consider blood-letting necessary, except in the rarest cases, ancient as well as medieval professors of medicine believed that they could under no circumstances dispense with it; in fact, it is probable that until the seventeenth century there was scarcely any form of disease the treatment of which would have been possible without withdrawal of blood. An actual system of blood-letting had been elaborated under the influence of humoro-pathological opinions. Every vein that could be reached with the lancet was acted upon, and the school of medicine of the period was punctiliously careful in teaching which vessel presented the most suitable point of attack for the hand of the physician in this or that form of disease. The therapeutic subtleties which were thus brought to light are beyond description. Thus, a withdrawal of blood from veins on the right side of the body was said to yield an essentially different effect from left-sided venesection, and each individual vein of the body promised a special advantage which was peculiar to this one vein. The physician of that period surely had enough to do to bear in mind all the numerous therapeutic effects which he was to achieve by the opening of the various veins. To facilitate this difficult art to a certain degree special figures were designed—so-called venesection manikins, in which the numerous points for bleeding were most carefully annotated. Fig. 5 (page 175) shows such a picture. It indicates no less than 53 different localities for venesection, and as each and every one of them again implied four or five, or possibly even more, methods of blood-letting, we may consider that there were many hundreds of different possibilities for phlebotomy. If it was easy to become lost in the labyrinth of this blood-thirsty therapy, the difficulty of a methodical application of venesection was very materially increased by astrology; for astrology differentiated between, first, favorable, then doubtful, and, finally, unfavorable days for venesection, basing this opinion upon certain positions between sun, moon, and planets. Then the various ages of life had also different days for venesection; days, for instance, which promised to be exceptionally successful for venesection in the young, offered very unfavorable prospects to the aged. Thus, for instance, the period from the first quadrature of the moon to the opposition was said to be excellent for bleeding in adolescence, whereas this period was by no means inviting for phlebotomy in those who had reached the senile period. The chances for venesection became rather intricate in their different aspects. Thus, for instance, Stöffler taught:

Conjunction of the moon with	the sun prohibits venesection two days before and one day after.
	Saturn Mars prohibits venesection one day before and one day after.
Quadrature of the moon with	Sun Saturn Mars prohibits venesection twelve hours before and twelve hours after.
Opposition of the moon with	Sun Saturn Mars prohibits venesection one day before and one day after.

We see, therefore, that the physician of that time was compelled to be well-versed in astronomy unless he meant to commit grave mistakes against the doctrines of *Medicina Astrologica*. Such sins could eventually become rather dangerous to the physician, for the code of Hammurabi (about 2200, B.C., ruler of Babylon) threatens the operator, for not quite unobjectionable surgical procedures, with the loss of his hands (Winckler, page 33, § 218).

In order to satisfy the astrological requirement of the physician most thoroughly, there arose in the middle ages a very peculiar literature. Under the name of an almanac or calendarium, thick folio volumes appeared, which enumerated, in long tables, the various positions of the planets and of the signs of the zodiac, so that the astrologer was enabled to note the fate of mankind rapidly and easily. The contents of such calendaria are beyond description. Apart from remarks which referred to all occurrences of civil life, was stated the exact period when to have the hair cut, when venesection was to be performed, when to draw teeth, when to take a bath, etc. Even the proper time for prayer was indicated by such a calendarium. According to the experience of Peter of Abano, the conjunction of the moon with Jupiter in the Dragon was sure to effect an answer to prayer. Hieronymus Cardanus had discovered, with the aid of astrology, that a request was sure to be complied with if a prayer was offered to the Virgin Mary on the first day of April, at 8 A.M. (Möhsen, Vol. II., page 423). Physicians excelled in the compilation of such calendaria, especially during the fifteenth and sixteenth centuries. Professors, forensic physicians, surgeons—in fact, all representatives of medical art—were equally intent upon instructing the public by calendaria in regard to the most various branches of *Medicina Astrologica*; thus, for instance, David Herliz, physician at Prenzlau, supplied Pomerania, Mecklenburg, and the Margravate of Brandenburg with calendars for fifty years, from the year 1584. The Marburg professor of medicine, Victorinus Schönfelder, played a similar rôle during the same period for western Germany. The physician, as almanac-maker, is probably one of the most wonderful results of medical superstition, and this aberration of medicine clung so firmly to the people that, even in the eighteenth and nineteenth centuries, certain days of the year were considered as especially favorable for venesection, and the calendars took particular pains to call the attention of the public most emphatically to good days for blood-letting.

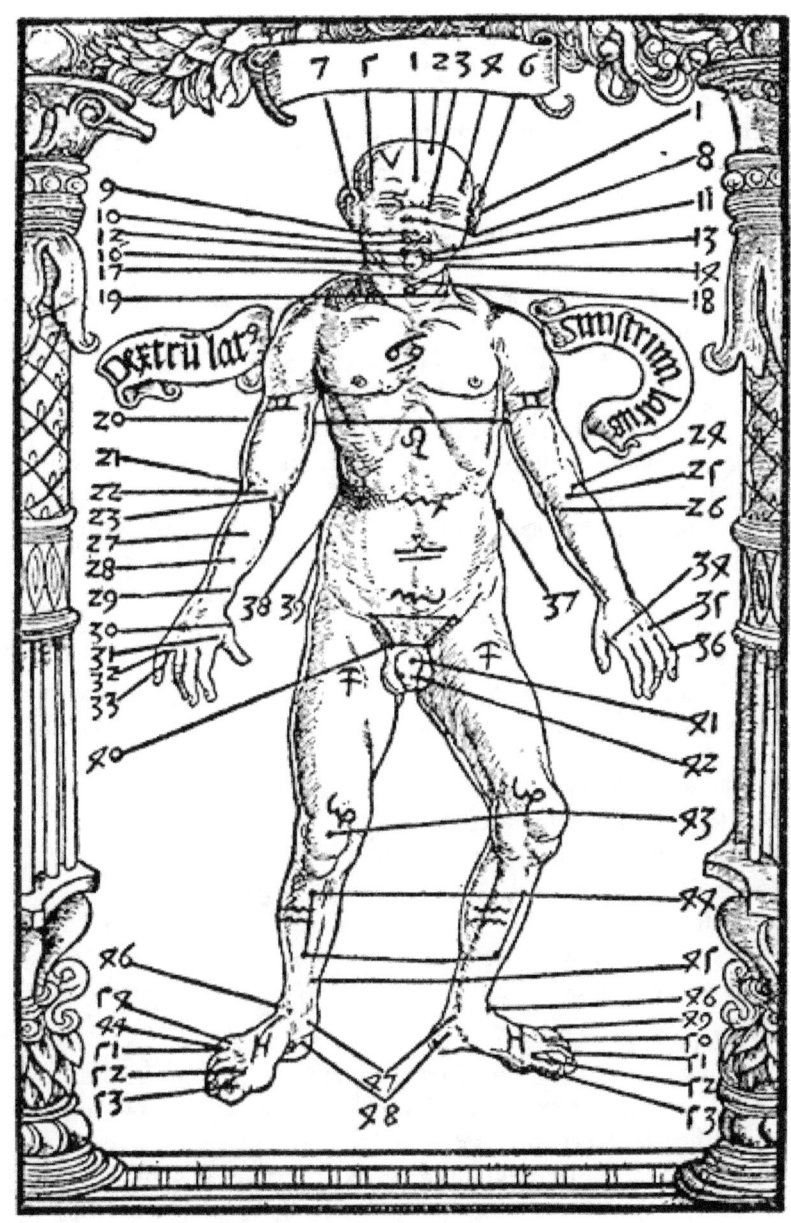

FIG. 5—VENESECTION IN ITS ASTRONOMICAL CONNECTION

Explanation of Fig. 5

A. The astronomic signs which are noted on the different parts of the body indicate the signs of the zodiac, under the special influence of which the respective members of the body are said to be.

B. The numerals which are found at the most varied parts of the body refer to indications for venesection, as stated below. In these localities, which are characterized by figures, blood was drawn for the most various affections, namely in:

- 1. Pains of the eyes and head; affections of the face, including eruptions.
- 2. Affections of the head; mental disturbances.
- 3. Affections of the eye of various kinds.
- 4 and 5. Pains in the ears; lachrymation.
- 6 and 7. Tinnitus aurium; tremor of the head.
- 8. Disturbances of hearing.
- 9. Heaviness of the head; flow from the eyes. Venesection here also renders memory more acute, as well as the activity of the brain in general.
- 10. Heaviness of the head.
- 11. Ulcers of the lips and of the gums.
- 12. The veins of the palate are to be opened in eruptions in the face, in toothache, in affections of the palate and of the mouth, heaviness of the head.
- 13. Neuralgia and toothache.
- 14. Headaches, mental disturbances.
- 15. To render the memory more acute.
- 16. In all affections of the mouth or of the chest.
- 17. Fetid breath.
- 18. Pains in the jaws; fœtor e naso; eruptions of the face.
- 19. Neuralgia of the head; eruptions.[175] [176]
- 20. Disturbances in the chest of various kinds.
- 21. Flow from the eyes; headache; epilepsy.
- 22. Diseases of the chest of various kinds, including dyspnea; headache; stitches in the side.
- 23. Diseases of the liver, injuries to the right side of the body; nosebleed.
- 24. Affections of the head and the eyes; pains in the shoulder-blades; coryza.
- 25. Pains in the heart, in the sides, and in the mouth.

- 26. Spasms in the fingers; pains in the spleen and in the limbs; epistaxis; stitches in the liver.
- 27. Pains of the central parts of the body.
- 28. Affections of the lower portions of the body.
- 29. Heart-disease.
- 30. To render vision more acute, and to strengthen the dexterity of the body.
- 31. Headache, fever, various kinds of cataract, glaucoma, etc.; cloudiness of the sclera; inflammations of the tongue and of the pharynx.
- 32. Pains of the head, lungs, spleen.
- 33. Diseases of the blood; chlorosis; jaundice; affections of the head; stitches in the right side. Blood-letting in this locality purifies liver, spleen, breast.
- 34. Same as 32.
- 36. Affections of the spleen, meningeal inflammation; hemorrhoids; stitches in the left side; renal affections; dysmenorrhea.
- 37. Affections of the spleen and of the bladder.
- 38. Dropsy; disturbances of digestion; ulcers of long standing.
- 39. Melancholia; venesection in this locality strengthens the kidneys.[177]
- 40. Hemorrhoids; strangury; disturbances of digestion; affections of the bladder and of the sexual organs.
- 41. Venesection here acts upon the proper condition of the body in general.
- 42. Diseases of the kidney, bladder, stone, testicles.
- 43. Venesection here strengthens the gait.
- 44. All kinds of pains of the lower extremities, such as arthritis, gout; also in dysmenorrhea.
- 45. Affections of the sexual organs; diseases of the kidney and bladder.
- 46. Diseases of the testicles.
- 47. Disturbances of menstruation; sterility of women; affections of the bladder and spleen.
- 48. Various kinds of diseases of the feet.
- 49. Dysmenorrhea; eruptions in the face and on the legs.
- 50. Apoplexy; paralysis.
- 51. Ophthalmia; skin diseases; cough; oppression of the chest.
- 52. Dysmenorrhea; affections of the testicles; costal pains.
- 53. Ophthalmia; dysmenorrhea; amenorrhea; skin eruptions.

Such therapy, detached entirely from the actual requirements of the case and based only upon observation of the sky, was bound to be attended with the most unfortunate results. The suffering public was frequently but little cheered by the assistance of its physicians, and often felt the desire to find out what another physician could do. It appears that such a condition occurred quite frequently, for Ptolemy, in number 57 of his "Centiloquium," gives special directions under what astral conditions such a change of physician could take place. He says: *"Cum septimum locum atque ejus dominum in ægritudine afflictum videris, medicum mutato."* It appears certain, accordingly, that a general change of physicians was inaugurated by the public so soon as the above conjunction was noted in the sky.

Those who desired to be very careful in the choice of their physician did not change only when the conjunction of the stars recommended it as advisable, but they also attempted to ascertain the horoscope of the newly chosen medical adviser, for medical wisdom was found in greatest abundance in a man whose aspects showed a certain form. *"Perfectus medicus erit, cui Mars et Venus fuerint in sexta,"* says Almansor.

This condition of *Astrologia Medica* was such as to weigh like an oppressive nightmare upon mankind, not only for centuries but for thousands of years, and in this way medical superstition has slaughtered more human beings than the most bloody wars ever did.

However, astrology has not always ruled our kind with equal strength. There were periods during which belief in the fate-determining power of the stars was more dominant, and others in which it was feebler. The ancient world, which was blindly devoted to all kinds of superstition, had also cherished and fostered astrology. But when the ancient theory of life was demolished later on, and the Christian God of love had taken possession of the world, the belief in the fate-determining power of the stars was shaken, and centuries, followed during which *Medicina Astrologica*, altho it did not by any means disappear entirely, was forced more or less to the rear. Astrology did not become resurrected until scholasticism and dogmatism had held back the activity of the mind from independent investigation, thus bringing about the intellectual darkness which for centuries prevailed. This use of astrology truly forms one of the most wonderful pages in the history of the development of our race, for an actual *furor astrologicus* seized upon the world in the course of the thirteenth century. The movement originated at the court of Emperor Frederick II. The great Ghibelline was so positive and so enthusiastic an adherent of all astrologic doctrines that he did not decide upon any undertaking until he had first learned the opinion of the stars regarding his enterprise. It was his firm belief that the stars prophesied for him a political rôle which was to shake the entire world, and of his astrological prediction he apprised his adversary, the pope, in the following words:

Fata volunt, stellaeque docent, animumque volatus,Quod Fridericus ego malleus orbis ero.

But if a ruler of high mental gifts is always destined to exert a powerful influence upon his epoch, how much more telling is this influence when the contemporaries of such a monarch lead a mental life, fettered by so many religious, philosophical, and physical prejudices as undeniably dominated mankind during the reign of the great Hohenstaufen. If these conditions were of the greatest advantage to astrology in general, circumstances shaped themselves most favorably for *Medicina Astrologica* in particular. Very soon after the death of the star-learned Hohenstaufen emperor, two highly talented physicians bound themselves body and soul to astrology—namely, Arnald Bachuone, called also, after his birthplace, Villanueva, Arnaldus Villanovanus or Arnald of Villanova (1235-1312), and Petrus, called also, after his birthplace, Abano near Padua, Petrus de Apono or Petrus Aponensis (1250-1315). From that time until the seventeenth century the most eminent representatives of all the sciences and professions devoted themselves to the doctrines of astrology. In the excellent work of Sudhoff is cited a notable number of physicians—by no means the most unskilful of their day—who confessed themselves to be iatromathematicians (i.e., *medici astrologici*). Astrology, and with it *Medicina Astrologica*, reigned supreme at most of the princely courts from the thirteenth to the seventeenth centuries. The Hohenstaufen, Frederick II., was, as we have seen, an implicit adherent to astrologic doctrines; likewise the Visconti in Milan. The royal court of Aragon in Palermo offered a sheltering asylum to astronomy and to astrology. Alfonso X. of Castile was so enthusiastic a friend of scientific astronomy that he ordered the planet-tables of Ptolemy to be restored, with an outlay of enormous costs, by fifty astronomers called by him to Toledo. German princes, such as Elector Joachim of Brandenburg, Albrecht, Elector of Mayence, Landgrave William of Hesse, Duke Albrecht of Prussia, not only adhered to the predictions of the stars, but they also subscribed to the statements of astrological medicine. Thus, for instance, Thomas Erastus (died 1583) the well-known opponent of Paracelsus, tells us that, as body-physician to the reigning count of Henneberg, he was not permitted to begin a course of treatment until he had consulted the stars. The German emperor, Charles V., was quite as constant a friend of the astrologists; he was instructed in astrology by his teacher, the subsequent pope, Hadrian VI. The court of Denmark was the center of astrological teachings under Frederick II., as no less a personage than Tycho de Brahe was active there. But not only rulers favored astrology, it met with implicit belief from highly enlightened scholars, statesmen, and naturalists. Thus, Melanchthon was so convinced an adherent of all astrological doctrines that he was incessantly active in their favor by mouth and by pen. And when fatal disease had finally seized upon him, he was soon satisfied as to the issue, in that Mars and Saturn happened to be in conjunction (Möhsen, Vol. II., page 416).

However, men were not wanting who courageously took up the battle against astrological delusions. Thus, for instance, the friend of Lorenzo of Medici, the learned Count Pico of Mirandola (1463-1494); also Girolamo Fracastori (1483-1553), who is known by his didactic poem on syphilis, opposed astrology.

If we now ask how it was possible that a superstition like astrology could for centuries dominate Occidental medicine, and was even able to influence the best minds in its favor, an answer to this question will not be as difficult as might appear at first glance. The very best and the most enlightened minds are always particularly affected by what is enigmatical and mysterious in the phenomena of life. They perceive the narrow limits set to our cognition of nature much more acutely and deeply than the average mind. This consciousness of the insufficiency of our own knowledge, joined with an ardent desire after a broadening of our understanding, tends to turn the mind in strange directions. The result of clearer self-knowledge in this modern epoch of ours is an adverseness to any form of romantic fancy, and is likely to end in a sad resignation that may result in pessimism. But the middle ages, with their exuberant confidence and faith, their belief in wonders, and their romantic ideas, did not suffer to any great extent from scientific apathy. A sharply defined, mystic tendency helped to overcome what was inadequate in the cognition of nature. And for this reason do we find this mystic tendency prominent, especially in those representatives of that period who, owing to their mental capacity, were bound to perceive their defective insight into the manifestations of life much more intensely than this was felt by the average persons of narrower intellect.

The conditions thus described, as well as the diagnostico-theoretical principles on which medicine and natural sciences were based in antiquity and in the middle ages, until late in the eighteenth century led many mentally gifted men to consider astrology rather a refuge from the current defective conception of natural phenomena than a false doctrine.

VI

INFLUENCE EXERTED UPON THE DEVELOPMENT OF SUPERSTITION BY MEDICINE ITSELF

AS ANCIENT, medieval, and some more modern theories of medicine have traveled over the same diagnostico-theoretical roads as did the natural science of those periods, they were naturally subject to the same errors and aberrations. But the consequences of their errors differed materially. Whereas natural science, in the early and middle ages, with its faulty diagnostico-theoretical method, too frequently had recourse to supernatural factors to explain terrestrial phenomena, and thus created superstition instead of elucidation, the pathology of ancient as well as of medieval medicine avoided as much as possible any recourse to miraculous agencies in explaining the pathological phenomena of the body. This it was forced to do for the sake of self-preservation. For what would have become of the physicians with their art, which was of a purely material kind, working as it did with drug and knife, if they themselves had traced disease to supernatural causes? No one, under such conditions, would have had any dealings with mundane medical science. It is true, there have been times when such a state of things actually existed. The physician, with his earthly appliances, was always led astray as soon as metaphysical ideas had victoriously entered pathology. History affords numerous examples of this. The cult of relics, the belief in astrology during half of the middle ages, show plainly to what a degrading position the physician was reduced as soon as a pathology reckoning with earthly factors was replaced by a metaphysical theory of disease. Then the physician was either completely thrust aside— ἀλλ᾽ ὠθεῖται μὲν ἔξω νοσοῦντος ὁ ἰατρός, as says Plutarch ("Superstition," Vol. I., page 412)—or he was forced to submit to a disgraceful interference. All schools of medicine, therefore, from the humoral pathology of the followers of Hippocrates to the so-called parasitism of the nineteenth century, have avoided as much as possible the acknowledgment that supernatural influences were active as pathological factors. Various as the principles of the countless medical schools may have been, they were all united in assuming as the starting-point of their speculations some material process of the body itself, in accordance with which they applied their therapeutic agencies.

Sometimes, it is true, it would seem as tho medicine, under some circumstances, had recourse to supernatural factors in explaining various phenomena of physiological as well as pathological conditions; as, for instance, in the primeval pneuma-doctrine, or in those conceptions which attribute to a mental or psychical principle a far-reaching influence upon the performance of all bodily functions. Upon closer investigation, however, we shall find that the pneuma, or spirit, the soul, or whatever else the mysterious mainspring of all phenomena of life may be called, was by no means conceived of by medicine as immaterial or supernatural. On the contrary!

159

Medicine, as often as it required a spiritual something to explain the manifestations of the body, has always regarded this unknown quantity as thoroughly substantial. It has not, indeed, been possible to determine more precisely the material nature of this great unknown, altho such attempts are by no means wanting in Democritus, Galen, and others; still it was always considered a corporeal thing. Supernatural qualities were ascribed to it only after death, but so long as the soul animated the body, united with the latter, it was a terrestrial being, and as such obeyed the laws of terrestrial substance. It was possible for medical science, therefore, to reckon with it in the explanation of pathological processes without necessarily expecting a reproach that supernatural agencies were called in for assistance.

Medicine, therefore, altho it has traveled the same diagnostico-theoretical road as natural science, has not, like the latter, directly produced superstition. It is true, it has called forth innumerable erroneous hypotheses. But a wrong hypothesis, altho it may be nonsensical to the utmost and give rise to the most serious practical consequences, is by no means superstition; for both error and superstition—so far as it is a question of medical matters—are two radically different conceptions, because the former concerns itself only with natural, the latter with supernatural factors.

Yet it is quite conceivable that the dissemination of an intellectual principle can be furthered and promoted without overt advocacy of the principle itself, and this was the relation that existed for thousands of years between medicine and superstition; for we learn from this investigation that the representatives of medicine were too often ready to admit all kinds of superstitious views into medicine. Whenever religion, philosophy, and natural science have seriously attempted to influence medicine in a manner promoting superstition, medical science yielded to these attempts, and this is the only reproach which can be justly laid at the door of our science.

However, this reproach is mitigated if we consider that medicine did not accord a home to superstition of its own free will, or even from a predilection for the heresies of other disciples, but it did so under compulsion; for the religious, the philosophical, the physical views which forced the entrance of superstition into medical science were almost always the views of a formidable party. It is a fact sufficiently demonstrated by history that powerful and far-reaching predilections of the popular mind resistlessly hurry along whatever is in their path. Such mental currents are the products of their period; they are the immediate result of the general sentiment and feeling of their time, and for this very reason they successfully overcome resistance. The opinion of a single individual may raise a protest against the spirit of the age, but this resistance is always bound to be in vain. The opinion of a single individual, even if it actually represents the truth, is absolutely powerless to resist the spirit of the age which, with elemental force, compels obedience. Therefore, the courageous, truth-seeking resistance which wasoffered to the heresies of *Medicina Astrologica* by Pico of Mirandola and Girolamo Fracastori was bound to be futile, because astrology was a genuine child of its time, and therefore held irresistible sway over thought and sentiment.

If religion and philosophy so often interfered with the development of medicine, this was only possible because the general tendency of the contemporary mind was thoroughly absorbed in this or that religious or philosophical idea. For each domain of human activity must needs be a mere reflection of the tendency which guides the mind of its period. This is a law which, with iron force, dominates the development of culture. Superstition in medicine, therefore, was bound to flourish and thrive whenever it harmonized with the spirit of the age.

This law, tho it may have checked the development of our science, nevertheless holds out the certain promise of a period, the intellectual power of which will thoroughly clear away all relics of superstition, which, still persisting in the minds of the many, drives them to the faith-curist and to the quack.

VII

MEDICAL SUPERSTITION AND INSANITY

THE history of medicine is conjoined with the evolution of theology to an extent which makes them almost inseparable, and this may best be seen from a study of the management of the insane, which is a continuous record of cruelty based upon medico-theological superstition. Perhaps the most heartrending chapter of unphilosophical theology teems with the narration of thousands of unfortunate beings murdered, tortured, and mishandled by the finesse in the interpretation of Biblical texts. The greatest triumph of modern medicine has consisted in unfettering the views of effete centuries, born of superstition and misconception, and in placing the treatment of the insane upon a humane, often even a curative, plane. As other afflictions of humanity were attributed to the agency of evil spirits, this was particularly the case with insanity; for if the evil one found it an easy task to control the corporeal acts of humanity, his power over the mental functions of the person afflicted was even greater. Hence, it was not the person who acted, but the evil spirit in him. Thus, the devil and his minions were the specific pathogenic agents.

This conception was not universal, for history shows us that clear thinkers, far in advance of their times, had an almost correct view of the nature of insanity—namely, that it was due to an affection of the mind. Among such men were Hippocrates,

Aretæus, Soranus, Galen, Aurelianus, etc., and some of the Mohammedan physicians. These apostles of science taught that insanity was a disease of the brain, and the most efficient remedy, mild, palliative treatment.

The belief which had flourished in most of the Oriental religions from remote antiquity, that the power of evil demons was the active cause of disease, particularly that lunacy was due to diabolic possession, became rooted in the early Christian Church and flourished for eighteen centuries, each leaf of this malignant plant representing countless unfortunates sacrificed to superstition. Later it was thought that the moon had a direct influence upon perturbation of the mind; hence, the term "lunacy" developed.

These doctrines gained special credence in the first centuries after Christ by the dissemination under the Church Fathers of the story of the miracles which they claimed had been performed by Jesus of Nazareth. Did not the Savior cast out devils? Did He not cure madness? The very word "epilepsy" shows by its derivation, ἐπίληψις (to seize upon), that possession was the presumable nature of the malady.

The noble work accomplished by the "pagan" pioneer alienists was discredited or forgotten, and the Church originated a process by which the possessed were to be treated. This method of treatment was derived purely from theologic sources, tempered with sufficient dogma. At first the treatment was gentle, in accordance with the spirit of the great physicians of antiquity, and if the afflicted one was not violent he was permitted to attend public worship. Sacred salves and holy water, the breath or the spittle of the officiating priest, the touching of relics, or a visit to holy places, were the principal therapeutic agents employed. These methods, even if they did no good (sometimes merely the consolation of a kind word from the priest had a beneficial effect), certainly did no harm, even tho such practises were factors in the spread of superstition.

This mild form of treatment did not, however, long continue. Soon measures were directed toward driving out the evil spirit from the possessed. This was attempted in various ways; first, by exorcism, in the period of Justin Martyr, and continued up to almost recent times (see Lecky, "History of European Morals"). "From the time of Justin Martyr for about two centuries, there is, I believe, not a single Christian writer who does not solemnly and explicitly assert the reality and frequent employment of this power."

One of the chief attributes of the devil was pride, therefore attempts were made by exorcism to pierce this vulnerable point in the armor of the evil one, and the foulest, vilest epithets were used to attain this end. It is impossible to-day to print these expressions, even in a work of scientific character, and it is better, perhaps, to refer such as are especially interested in them to the *Manuale Benedictionum*, by the Bishop of Passau, published in 1849, and similar works. Adjuvants to this form of treatment consisted in "frightening" the devil by long words, difficult to pronounce, commonly derived from Oriental languages, by the administration of malodorous and filthy "drugs," and similar practises.

It was claimed that many devils were thus driven out, and the annals of the Church contain numerous records of persons cured in this manner. "The Jesuit Fathers at Vienna, in 1583, glorified in the fact that in such a contest they had cast out twelve thousand, six hundred and fifty-two living devils" (White). The prevalence of these ideas to such a degree in the minds of the people may be noted from the fact that, in the churches themselves, such scenes are carved in stone and depicted on canvas. Medieval drama teemed with similar conceptions, and this condition of affairs prevailed for over one thousand years, unfortunately not in this harmless manner, but supplemented by great cruelty, which forms, perhaps, the most terrible chapter in the history of medical superstition.

The subtleties of theologic interpretation soon evolved a more comprehensive method of dealing with the "possessor" and the possessed. As an appeal to pride was ineffectual and noxious drugs unavailing, it was found necessary to whip the devil out, or the unfortunate individuals were imprisoned, and as a refinement of this treatment they were even tortured. Thus the jailer for a long time played the part of a specialist in lunacy, with the clergy in consultation. Places in which the insane were confined were known as "fool towers" and "witch towers."

This state of things was not altered with the dawn of the Reformation. The writings of Luther conclusively show his ideas in regard to possession and witchcraft, and these views under Calvin reached enormous development. Even Cotton Mather, in many respects far in advance of his times, and who himself had known persecution, was not emancipated from these delusions, and Salem has many a story to tell of possession and witch-baiting. It is true we may quite properly consider these views as the thought of the times, but, in many other respects, Luther, Calvin, and Mather were in advance of their period, and, therefore, a justification for their actions is not quite apparent. Marcus Aurelius also was much superior to his age, yet was grateful to his teachers that they taught him to disregard superstition in all its various forms.

It is not unlikely that conditions of this kind frequently led to epidemics—if not of actual insanity, at least to hysteria—which not rarely developed in cities, nunneries, and monasteries; thus the epidemics in Erfurt in 1237, in the Rhine countries in 1374, and many others (see Hirsch).

It is rather remarkable that while such views and practises prevailed in the Christian Church, the followers of Mohammed not only held different views, but adopted a mode of treatment of the insane which laid the foundation of modern therapeutics in diseases of the mind. In the twelfth century, in Bagdad, a palace called the "Home of Mercy" was built, in which the insane were confined, examined every month, and released as soon as they had recovered. An asylum in Cairo was founded in 1304, while the first Christian asylum expressly for the mad is noted in 1409 (Lecky).

But science fought its way through the barriers of ignorance, misdirected zeal, and superstition. Altho there were physicians and "magicians," who conformed to the views of the Church, the seed sown by the earlier schools of medicine slowly but surely began to put forth shoots, and the result was a tree of knowledge, the fruit of which may be observed in every modern insane asylum of the world, where the unfortunate sufferer is treated with kindness and skill, which, fortunately, often results in cure.

Scientific reason frequently rebelled against the "insane superstition," at first mildly, but constantly increasing in strength, until an effectual protest was finally raised by John Weir, of Cleves, who was soon followed by Michel de Montaigne. And now a battle royal was waged between the adherents of theology and the disciples of the "resurrected" truth, and once more in the history of the world was demonstrated the correctness of the saying, that "truth crushed to earth shall rise again." All over the world the warfare was carried, and at the end of the eighteenth century new champions arose—Jean Baptiste Pinel in France, and William Tuke in England. Their followers are legion, and in the book of life, in letters of gold, many a name has been written of those who trod in the footsteps of these pioneers. Theology no longer interferes in the treatment of the insane; in fact, it would be manifestly unjust not to mention that many Christian theologians subsequently joined in the noble work of lunacy reform, and aided progress greatly.

How great this progress in the treatment of the insane can best be appreciated by some of the older physicians in practise to-day. Who does not remember the chains, the strait-jacket, the dark locked cells of the insane asylum? These conditions existed not very many years ago, and altho the novels of Charles Reade are no doubt greatly exaggerated in regard to the conditions he portrayed in insane asylums, yet *more than a grain of truth* is probably contained in them. The books did much to bring about reforms in England and elsewhere.

Modern alienists have wrought wonders; their successful operations are not published in the daily press, but any visitor who knows what an insane asylum was fifty years ago, and who spends a few hours in a modern hospital for the treatment of lunatics, will observe what appears but little short of the miraculous. Imagine two thousand or more insane persons dining in a large hall, upon the table a tablecloth, and the insane using knife and fork in a decorous manner, and when the visitor is told that the "violent ward" is also present, and is asked to single these out from among the many, and fails (as he invariably does), the results attained by science, above all other measures, are strikingly apparent.